北京市自然科学基金项目成果（Z200016）

中国医学科学院医学与健康科技创新工程重大协同项目成果（2021-I2M-1-056）

动脉粥样硬化性脑血管病

本体构建与知识组织

主　编　李子孝　李　姣

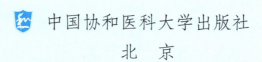

中国协和医科大学出版社

北　京

图书在版编目（CIP）数据

动脉粥样硬化性脑血管病本体构建与知识组织 / 李子孝, 李姣主编. -- 北京：中国协和医科大学出版社, 2024. 9. -- ISBN 978-7-5679-2478-9

Ⅰ. R743

中国国家版本馆CIP数据核字第20240T6V53号

主　　编　李子孝　李　姣
责任编辑　李元君　胡安霞
封面设计　邱晓俐
责任校对　张　麓
责任印制　黄艳霞
出版发行　中国协和医科大学出版社
　　　　　（北京市东城区东单三条9号　邮编100730　电话010-65260431）
网　　址　www.pumcp.com
印　　刷　小森印刷（北京）有限公司
开　　本　710mm×1000mm　1/16
印　　张　15.75
字　　数　290千字
版　　次　2024年9月第1版
印　　次　2024年9月第1次印刷
定　　价　78.00元

编者名单

主　　编　李子孝　李　姣

编　　者　李子孝　李　姣　马鹤桐　沈　柳

　　　　　王嘉阳　王春娟　杨　林　陈子墨

　　　　　徐晓巍　王　孟　王序文　闫　然

前　言

　　动脉粥样硬化性脑血管病是导致中老年人残疾和死亡的重要病因之一，随着我国人口老龄化趋势的加剧，该疾病的发病率呈现逐年上升的趋势，给社会和家庭带来了沉重的负担。面对这一严峻形势，加强该疾病的基础研究、提高临床诊疗水平及完善疾病管理体系具有重要意义。本体构建与知识组织作为一种有效的智能技术，可以为动脉粥样硬化性脑血管病的研究和防治提供有力支持。通过本体构建，可以对该疾病的相关概念、症状、病因、病理、诊断、治疗和预防等方面的知识进行系统化组织，便于进行计算机处理和智能推理。此外，本体可以实现不同学科领域、研究人员之间的资源共享和交流，提高研究效率。

　　尽管动脉粥样硬化性脑血管病的发病率及危害性较高，但目前社会对于该疾病的关注度仍然不足，也缺乏针对该疾病的统一认知。为了更好地认识该疾病，组织、整合和分析相关的生物医学知识，需要构建动脉粥样硬化性脑血管病知识框架并明确范围。构建动脉粥样硬化性脑血管病本体旨在为生物医学研究提供一个结构化的、标准化的知识框架，以促进对该疾病的理解、研究及临床应用。通过构建本体整合来自不同领域（如病理学、影像学、分子生物学等方面）的研究成果，形成一个统一的知识体系，提供一种共同的、标准化的语言，使得不同研究团队、不同研究机构之间可以更加顺畅地进行学术交流和信息共享，帮助研究者快速找到相关的研究数据和成果，提高研究的效率，挖掘疾病与基因、药物、生物标志物等之间的关系，从而促进新知识的发现，为临床医生提供决策支持，以及作为教育工具帮助学生和研究人员更好地了解疾病的复杂性和研究的最新进展。动脉粥样硬化性脑血管病本体的构建可以在生物医学研究、药物发现、临床诊断和治疗、流行病学研究、生物信息学工具研发、教育培训、知识共享与交流、科研资源整合、知识发现的过程中起到支撑的作用。

　　本书旨在系统介绍动脉粥样硬化性脑血管病本体的构建与知识组织方法，内容包括该疾病的背景与意义、相关研究、构建流程、结构设计、数据统计、审核机制、结果评估、扩展应用等，本体部分涵盖临床表现、诊断、治疗、危险因素、病理生理、康复预防等内容。为了与国际接轨，主要知识框架和部分术语参照脑卒中本体（STO），在其基础上进行调整与扩展，并进行了中英文术语的补充和对齐，以驱动大语言模型开展知识发现等具体应用。为了更加全面准确地覆盖动脉粥样硬化性脑血管病本体的内容与范围，术语收集来自不同词表、本体、术语集等，尽可能扩充多种表达方式。由于该本体为初次汇编，涉及内容广泛，难免存在一些不足。随着动脉粥样硬化性脑血管病诊疗技术的不断提高，该本体已发布在国际生物本体共享平台 Bioportal 上，研究团队会持续做好更新工作。

　　最后，衷心感谢参与本书编写的各位专家、学者及学会的大力支持！

李子孝　李　姣

2024年6月

目　录

第一章

绪　论

第一节　动脉粥样硬化性脑血管病本体构建背景与意义

动脉粥样硬化性脑血管病是引起绝大多数缺血性脑卒中的主要原因，该疾病常导致患者死亡或残疾[1]。尽管动脉粥样硬化性脑血管病发病率高，危害性强，但目前尚无针对该疾病的明确边界或详尽的统计数据。此前，一项研究将动脉粥样硬化性脑血管病定义为"缺血性脑卒中和短暂性缺血性发作"的集合[2]，表明动脉粥样硬化性脑血管病与脑卒中之间密不可分的联系。脑卒中是全球第二大死亡原因和成人身体残疾的主要原因，其中缺血性脑卒中占所有脑卒中的87%[3-6]。在美国，每年有超过79.5万人遭遇脑卒中，其中61万人是首次发病，18.5万人有过脑卒中经历[6-7]。每年大约有14万人因脑卒中去世，占美国总死亡人数的1/5左右，使其成为美国的第五大死因[3-6]。美国每年因脑卒中产生的医疗费用、药物开销及工作损失总计约340亿美元[7]。脑卒中后可能出现的神经功能缺陷包括平衡问题、偏瘫、感觉和振动觉丧失、麻木、反射减弱、上睑下垂、视野缺损、失语和失用症[8-11]。全球范围内，每年有约4400万人因脑卒中而残疾，并有约550万人因此死亡[5]。2011年，我国40岁以上人群中缺血性脑卒中的发病人数达到约133.4万。2012年，中国脑卒中的标化患病率约为1.82%，据此估算我国患者超过1000万例。此外，我国脑卒中疾病呈现年轻化趋势，65岁以下的患者约占一半[12]。1992—2014年，抽样调查显示我国首次脑卒中发病率为297/10万人，而且性别和脑卒中类型之间存在显著差异，总体增加了6.3%，男性增加了5.5%，女性增加了7.9%，出血性脑卒中增加了4.6%，而缺血性脑卒中增加了7.3%[13-14]。中国每年大约有2.5亿例新发脑卒中病例，并且这个数字还在增加[13-14]。尽管现代医学、药物和医疗技术的进步在一定程度上降低了脑卒中的病死率，但仍然给个人带来了较高的发病和死亡风险，给社会造成了巨大的经济负担。2000—2010年，美国的脑卒中相对死亡率下降了35.8%[15]，然而，每年仍有近80万美国人受到脑卒中的影响，许多幸存者在日常生活中面临持续的挑战[16]。在美国，超过2/3的脑卒中幸存者在住院后需要接受康复治疗[17]。尽管卒中中心的系统在不断改进以早期识别脑卒中症状并迅速提供治疗，但只有少数急性脑卒中患者能够接受溶栓治疗，许多患者仍然存在不同程度的功能缺陷[16]。

缺血性脑卒中是动脉粥样硬化性脑血管病的主要类型之一，全球缺血性脑卒中的发病率为101.3/10万人[18]。1993—2015年全球基于人群和医院研究的大型荟萃分析显示，缺血性脑卒中的主要亚型包括心脏栓塞、大动脉粥样硬化、小血管闭塞等，其中心脏栓塞占22%，大动脉粥样硬化占23%，小血管闭塞占22%[6,19]。缺血性脑卒中的亚型分布在不同种族或民族群体中可能有所不同[19]。溶栓治疗是缺血性脑卒中的唯一有效治疗方法，但由于大多数患者不符合溶栓标准，在脑卒中症状出现后4.5小时内进行溶栓治疗的患者不到5%[20]。因此，大多数脑卒中患者会有残余的神经功能缺损[21-22]。

随着动脉粥样硬化性脑血管病的发病率、致死率、致残率的增加，该疾病越来越受到重视。然而，目前国内外对该疾病的认知存在分歧，阻碍了研究的快速推进。为了满足医师、数据科学家、医学信息学科研人员对该疾病信息的需求，本研究构建动脉粥样硬化性脑血管病本体作为知识表示和知识共享的载体。本体是对现实世界的一部分的概念化表示，它通过类、关系、功能、个体和语义规则定义了一个共享话语领域的表征词汇。本体是构建语义模型的较好选择，允许包含人机可读的信息、来自逻辑描述谓词的定义，以及通过来自医疗记录和公理的信息进行推理。医学领域的本体意义深远，因为本体允许以完善的组织形式和清晰的方式交换从各种来源获得的信息，如书籍、文章、经验和专家的知识。本体构建完成后，也应积极应用于电子病历等临床密切相关的真实世界的数据中。电子病历内含许多丰富的临床数据，可以支持医疗处方、改善疾病管理，同时有助于减少严重的用药错误。随着以深度学习为代表的机器学习模型的涌现，这些海量数据亟待挖掘。而电子病历中的数据多为自由文本，利用自然语言处理技术将自由文本转换为结构化数据后才能实现对该类数据最好的利用。因此，本研究基于动脉粥样硬化性脑血管病实现本体构建，完成在该疾病涉及的内容的框架设计及概念填充，并完成概念的双语化表示，为涉及该疾病领域的工作人员提供明确的知识边界、知识组织及知识表示。

第二节 动脉粥样硬化性脑血管病本体相关研究

本研究对知识图谱、本体、词表等资源进行了调研，以可复用资源做基础，包括通用领域、医学领域、跨语种领域和神经疾病领域的资源。在通用领域中，目前已有大量知识图谱能够提供海量数据，如单语种的知识图谱，只能提供有限的借鉴。在跨语种领域中，许多已实现了双语构建的知识图谱，但支持中英双语的跨语种知识图谱中包含动脉粥样硬化性脑血管病的内容较少。相比之下，医学领域的本体、知识图谱等资源与目标内容更为贴近。医学领域本体及图谱集成资源，如词表、术语集等不仅可以提供框架设计参考，还可进行术语扩充。尽管医学领域的大量资源能为建设动脉粥样硬化性脑血管病提供大量方法基础，但在内容上，该疾病仍然比较特别，无法大量复用来自医学通用领域的内容作为基础。

在神经疾病领域中，我们同样调研了大量相关资源。其中，NeuroWeb 是涵盖脑血管疾病术语、表型、通用医学概念及临床指征的本体。Onto NeuroBase Ontology 是面向神经成像相关的领域本体，包括医学影像和医学影像处理工具。DStrokeOnto ontology 是针对脑卒中诊断和病患管理的本体。NeuMORE 是针对脑卒中后的恢复所开发的本体。神经系统疾病本体（neurological disease ontology）则是针对神经系统疾病和医学实践开发的本体。美国国立卫生研究院卒中量表本体（National Institutes of Health Stroke Scale Ontology）是针对脑卒中评估的临床表型开发的本体。神经系统检查本体(neurologic examination ontology)是面向神经系统检查方面的本体，其数据范围涵盖精神状态检查、运动能力检查、脑神经检查、感知能力检查、协调性检查、步态平衡检查、颈部检查、头部检查等，但疾病只包括肌张力障碍和帕金森病。脑卒中本体（the stroke ontology，STO）[23]是针对脑卒中开发的英文本体，内容涵盖生物医学及危险因素概念、预防、病因、病理生理学、生物标志物、合并症、并发症、诊断、治疗等内容。人体表型本体（human phenotype ontology，HPO）[24]是面向表型的本体，内容涵盖人类表型、医学相关表型、疾病表型等。多发性硬化症本体（multiple sclerosis ontology）是面向多发性硬化症的本体，内容涵盖临床特征，病因学，多发性硬化症的模型、通路的分子机制，分子和细胞特征，多发性硬化症的社会和经济影响，以及治疗等。其他相关本体包括阿尔茨海默病本体（Alzheimer disease ontology，ADO），帕金森病本体（Parkinson disease ontology，PDON），癫痫本体（epilepsy ontology）等面向某一特定疾病的本体。但以上资源中，部分未能公开使用，绝大多数本体由于其聚焦内容、组织形式、分类方法等方面无法被大量复用，但对开发动脉粥样硬化性脑血管病本体仍然提供了参考和借鉴。在调研的过程中，课题组选定 STO 作为主要参照本体，该本体涵盖脑卒中领域的主要生物医学和风险因素概念，并辅以同义术语、定义及参考来源，纳入不同人群的需求视角，其构建过程包括需求确定、知识获取、概念框架设计、信息整合与规范化、术语分析及概念扩充，以及本体评价，最终形成第一个在脑卒中领域的多视角本体，其可以作为多源异构数据的知识规范化表示。STO 分为八大顶层类，覆盖 1719 个概念，11 个层级，涵盖脑卒中诊断、治疗、预后的一系列概念。在构建动脉粥样硬化性脑血管病本体时，课题组选取STO作为主要本体参考框架，并借鉴其构建流程，在原本体复用的基础上实现了增删查改的操作。

第二章

动脉粥样硬化性脑血管病本体构建

第一节　本体构建流程

动脉粥样硬化性脑血管病本体是基于本体开发（ontology development）101[25]方法论和专家意见实现构建的，该本体构建流程包括以下9个步骤。

一、收集并明确临床需求

在这一步骤中，需要明确临床需求，构建的本体在多大程度上可以帮助解决问题，本体的目标是什么，以及如何评估有效性和必要性。从临床的角度来看，动脉粥样硬化性脑血管病是一种发病率高、界限不清、共识不明确的疾病。因此，以一种适当的方式，即本体，分享对这种疾病的现有认知是至关重要的。

二、背景调查和知识获取

在调研了本体建模、医学本体构建、跨语言资源等相关内容后，以本体开发101方法论为基础，借鉴多学科专家的宝贵经验，开发以动脉粥样硬化性脑血管病为重点的跨语种本体。构建的本体应涵盖疾病的主要方面，特别是临床表现。

三、本体复用

通过对现有本体的优缺点分析，决定复用STO。STO是针对脑卒中的最新本体，从多个角度涵盖了较为全面的医学概念。考虑到动脉粥样硬化性脑血管病与脑卒中范畴相互覆盖内容较多，STO的复用可以在较大程度上促进内容扩展和使用，为国际合作交流提供便利。

四、确定范围

STO 与所要构建的本体范畴并不相同。因此，需要对当前本体的整体框架进行修订，包括分支裁剪、概念删除或添加，以及临床医生评估。脑卒中类型包括缺血性脑卒中、出血性脑卒中、短暂性脑缺血发作等。动脉粥样硬化性脑血管病是缺血性脑卒中和短暂性脑缺血发作的一个集合。然而，STO 包含了大量来自不同脑卒中类型的概念。因此，有必要对 STO 进行适当的裁剪和修正以符合动脉粥样硬化性脑血管病的范畴。构建本体的过程中，邀请神经外科临床医生参与本体构建任务，并完成范畴确定的工作。

五、确定策略

经过与临床医生、数据科学家和本体专家的讨论，决定设计包括动脉粥样硬化性脑血管病临床表现、合并症、并发症、诊断、模型、发病机制、预防、康复、危险因素和治疗在内的十大顶级分类。本体增加了"康复"和"动脉粥样硬化性脑血管病分型"作为两个顶层类，因为无论罹患动脉粥样硬化性脑血管病的严重程度如何，康复都是该疾病恢复中不可缺少的重要环节，而治疗方案应根据对具体疾病分型的认识来确定。

六、概念提取

对现有康复资源的研究并未发现完整的康复术语、本体或分支可以复用，只有零星的术语是相关的。因此，分别查阅国内外康复相关指南和文献，并提取概要和详细目录，经3位具有医学信息学背景的专家讨论后对双语框架和内容进行调整，概念经审核后进行保留。康复类作为创建的顶层类之一，主要包括评估、装备、管理、类型4个方面，其具体概念从不同语言的医学指南中提取并对齐到本体中。

七、概念扩展

本环节在确定部分概念的基础上进行扩展，主要涉及以下几个方面。首先，由于临床诊断很大程度上依赖于临床特征，临床表现的概念需要扩展。在调研现有的以临床表现为中心的本体和术语后，选择HPO作为目标本体，将HPO中的分支扩展到当前本体。其次，当前本体中的术语有大量的同义术语需要进行扩充。具体来说，将每个概念与系统化临床医学术语集（systematized nomenclature of medicine--clinical terms，SNOMED CT）和国际疾病分类第11版（international classification of diseases 11th，ICD-11）中的对应概念进行映射，并将额外的同义词纳入本体中。对于没有映射结果，即没有完成同义词扩充的概念，同时邀请具有医学信息学背景的研究生加入并对每个概念进行了审编，选取适当的同义术语。

八、本体验证

本体验证需要多学科的专家共同进行，因此，邀请国内顶级医院脑卒中专科临床医生对本体进行审查。对两位专家提出不同结论的情况，邀请第三位专家介入。当第三位专家对术语无法确定时，将引入第四位专家进行共同审核。

九、本体评估

本体构建完成后，需要对其进行评估，以了解在真实世界中该本体是否能够为科研所用。为评估本体，首先，要对本体做统计，包括每个顶层类的概念数量、中文和英文术语数量等。其次，设定特定场景，在本方案中以文献分类为例，测定本体是否能够在文献分类方面起到支撑作用。

第二节　本体结构设计

动脉粥样硬化性脑血管病本体是一个结构化的知识框架，旨在整合和规范关于此类疾病的概念和信息。在医疗健康领域，本体的构建对于加强疾病信息的组织、促进跨语言检索、支持研究人员的知识发现，以及辅助临床决策具有重要意义。当前本体涵盖了动脉粥样硬化性脑血管病的核心概念，具体包括十个顶层类，分别是动脉粥样硬化性脑血管病的临床表现、合并症、并发症、诊断、模型、发病机制、预防、康复、危险因素和治疗。以下是顶层分类的内容，本体的结构设计见表1。

表 1　本体结构设计

中文	英文
危险因素	Risk factor
可改变的危险因素	Modifiable risk factors
不可改变的危险因素	Nonmodifiable risk factors
并发症	Complication
出血转化	Hemorrhagic transformation
出血性卒中	Hemorrhagic stroke
脑水肿	Cerebral edema
脑疝	Cerebral hernia
消化道出血	Gastrointestinal bleeding
肺炎	Pneumonia
泌尿系感染	Urinary tract infection
吞咽障碍	Dysphagia
压疮	Decubitus
深静脉血栓形成	Deep vein thrombosis
肺栓塞	Pulmonary embolism
心脏骤停	Cardiac arrest
心肌梗死	Myocardial infarction
癫痫发作	Epileptic seizure
合并症	Comorbidity
卒中前合并症	Prestroke comorbidity
共病措施	Comorbidity measures
卒中后合并症	Post-stroke comorbidity
动脉粥样硬化性脑血管病分型	**Classification of atherosclerotic cerebrovascular disease**
TOAST 分型	Trial of ORG 10172 in acute stroke treatment
中国缺血性卒中亚型	Chinese ischemic stroke subclassification
缺血性卒中分型系统亚型	Subtypes of ischemic stroke classification system
缺血性卒中病因分类系统	Causative classification system
治疗	**Treatment**
动脉粥样硬化性脑血管病的治疗	Treatment of atherosclerotic cerebrovascular disease
一般疗法	General treatment

中文	英文
康复	Rehabilitation
康复管理	Management of rehabilitation
康复类型	Types of rehabilitation
康复评价	Assessment of rehabilitation
康复设备	Equipment of rehabilitation
预防	Prevention
动脉粥样硬化性脑血管病的一级预防	Primary prevention of atherosclerotic cerebrovascular disease
动脉粥样硬化性脑血管病的二级预防	Secondary prevention of atherosclerotic cerebrovascular disease
发病机制	Pathogenesis
动脉粥样硬化性脑血管病的发病机制	Pathogenesis of atherosclerotic cerebrovascular disease
动脉粥样硬化性脑血管病的病理生理学	Pathophysiology of atherosclerotic cerebrovascular disease
临床表现	Clinical manifestation
小脑梗死综合征	Cerebellar infarction syndrome
椎基底动脉梗死综合征	Vertebrobasilar infarction syndrome
腔隙性脑梗死症状	Lacunar infarction syndrome
脉络膜前动脉梗死综合征	Anterior choroidal artery infarction syndrome
大脑前动脉梗死综合征	Anterior cerebral artery infarction syndrome
基底动脉梗死综合征	Basilar artery infarction syndrome
大脑半球梗死综合征	Hemispheric infarction syndrome
大脑后动脉梗死综合征	Posterior cerebral artery infarction syndrome
大脑中动脉梗死综合征	Middle cereberal artery infarction syndrome
颈内动脉梗死综合征	Internal carotid artery infarction syndrome
分水岭梗死综合征	Watershed infarction syndrome
脑干梗死综合征	Brainstem infarction syndrome
丘脑梗死综合征	Thalamic infarction syndrome
诊断	Diagnosis
诊断动脉粥样硬化性脑血管病的生物标志物	Biomarkers for the diagnosis of atherosclerotic cerebrovascular disease
鉴别诊断	Differential diagnosis
神经解剖	Neuroanatomy
神经传导通路	Nerve pathway
动脉粥样硬化性脑血管病评价	Evaluation of atherosclerotic cerebrovascular disease

一、临床表现

这一类别涵盖了动脉粥样硬化性脑血管病患者可能出现的各种症状和综合征，如大脑前动脉梗死综合征可能涉及无动性缄默症、行为障碍等多种临床表现。

二、合并症

这一类别分为普遍共病、卒中后共病和卒中前共病，涉及患者在动脉粥样硬化性脑血管病基础上可能出现的其他疾病，需要进行综合管理。

三、并发症

这一类别描述了动脉粥样硬化性脑血管病及其治疗过程中可能出现的各种并发症，如心搏骤停、吞咽困难等，这些并发症可能严重影响患者的预后。

四、诊断

这一类别包括生物标志物、脑部解剖学诊断、鉴别诊断及评估方法。这些诊断工具和标准对于准确识别疾病至关重要。

五、分型

这一类别涉及动脉粥样硬化性脑血管病的病理生理学和发病机制模型，有助于理解疾病的发展过程，为预防及治疗提供理论基础。

六、发病机制

这一类别深入探讨动脉粥样硬化性脑血管病的分子机制、生物学过程和社会环境因素，为揭示疾病的根本原因提供线索。

七、预防

这一类别涵盖一级预防和二级预防策略，旨在减少疾病的发生率和减轻严重程度，包括健康教育、饮食调整、药物治疗等。

八、康复

作为重点分支，这一类别涵盖了从评估到治疗的各种康复方法。康复评价不仅关注疾病相关的能力，也包括环境支持和康复需求评估。

九、危险因素

这一类别区分了可改变和不可改变的危险因素，为个体化治疗和预防策略提供了依据。

十、治疗

这一类别包括一般治疗（如血压控制、心脏监测）和针对动脉粥样硬化性脑血管病的特定治疗（如抗血小板药物、搭桥手术等）。

第三节　本体数据统计

对当前本体进行数据统计，表2显示了本体的概况，包括概念数量、顶层概念分支、中英术语数量、中英同义词数量和每个概念分支的中英定义数量。本体共有1719个概念，涵盖中文术语4589个，英文术语6621个。其中，临床表现类和诊断类包含的概念最多，占总概念的50%以上。临床表现中出现中英同义词最多，分别为742个和1153个，同时定义最多，包括中文定义172个，英文定义373个。康复概念数量位列其次，覆盖224个概念，中英术语分别为603个和1022个，中文定义为25个。康复作为一个全新的分支，无论是在本体还是在真实世界的治

表2　本体统计数据

概念分支	概念	中文术语	英文术语	中文同义词	英文同义词	中文定义	英文定义	层级
诊断	488	954	1442	466	953	8	219	8
临床表现	431	1173	1584	742	1153	172	373	9
康复	224	603	1022	379	798	25	0	6
发病机制	219	767	1059	548	840	0	78	11

续　表

概念分支	概念	中文术语	英文术语	中文同义词	英文同义词	中文定义	英文定义	层级
治疗	150	385	463	235	313	0	53	8
危险因素	126	516	735	390	609	0	32	9
预防	117	355	417	238	300	0	54	8
合并症	51	160	341	109	290	0	29	7
并发症	18	58	117	40	99	2	0	3
分型	5	6	18	1	13	0	2	2
去重总计	1719	4589	6621	2867	4901	197	774	11

疗路径中都发挥着不可或缺的作用。分型包含了5个概念，均为国际知名的分型。在所有概念中，超过20个术语的概念有23个，最多包含41个术语，超过10个术语的概念有307个。当前本体由多个层级组成，最深的层级达到11层，属于发病机制一类。60%的顶层类包含8个及以上层级，大多数概念可以在第4层级找到。具体的信息可以在表2中找到。

第四节　本体数据审核机制

由于本体数据的来源多样，包括STO的复用概念、对其他图谱或词表的映射、对中英指南的内容抽取以及人工标注与对齐，因此，需要对数据进行审核，尽可能地保证数据的准确。对本体数据的审核主要集中在以下方面：①术语范围确定，即一个概念是否属于动脉粥样硬化性脑血管病的范畴。②分支确定，即一个概念是否应该属于该细分分支。③术语准确性，即两种语言中的术语是否为该概念的同义词。④拼写错误，即一个术语是否有拼写错误。⑤术语重复，即一个术语是否在不适当的情况下出现。⑥语言错误，即在选择特定语言时是否出现语言错误。

第三章

动脉粥样硬化性脑血管病本体结果和应用

第一节 结果评估

本体的开发有助于对多源异构的健康数据进行知识整合，对数据进行标准化处理，并增强数据互操作性。面向特定领域的本体，如动脉粥样硬化性脑血管病本体，在知识标准化、知识集成、知识标注和知识表示等方面发挥着重要作用，并可以辅助临床决策支持。尽管动脉粥样硬化性脑血管病是一种高发疾病，但目前从业人员还未对该疾病涉及的医学知识达成共识，考虑到该疾病的重要性不容忽视，且其知识边界不清晰，因此，亟需设计开发涉及该疾病覆盖范围的本体。课题组通过范围确定、概念提取、框架搭建等流程构建了一个结构化的内容较为全面的动脉粥样硬化性脑血管病本体，供该领域的研究人员、专家和临床医生参考。

目前的本体主要由1719个概念、4589个中文术语和6621个英文术语组成。该本体根据临床需要进行深度扩展，实现康复本体设计，并提供跨语言术语内容。本体可以辅助实体识别，提供知识体系，进而辅助临床诊断和治疗。在本体构建完成后，课题组在本体覆盖范围、本体精确性、本体一致性、本体可扩展性、本体简洁性、本体易于理解性、本体互操作性、本体语义丰富性、本体实用性和本体功能性等方面分别邀请临床医生进行评估，并据此生成《动脉粥样硬化性脑血管病中英术语专家共识》。对于某一个具体的概念，用户可以通过打开发布在BioPortal上的层级结构进行筛选，也可以直接通过输入具体的概念进行检索，在本体界面上可以看到概念的中英文优选词、同义词，以及其所处的分支结构、定义及来源，见图1。

此外，在实用性方面，对于一线临床医生、科研人员来说，能够通过本体定位到合适的文献内容十分必要且有意义，因此设计文献分类的场景，并使用具体指标来评估本体在该场景下的实用性。课题组抽取动脉粥样硬化性脑血管病相关文献600篇，抽取文献标题及摘要，并选择最为常见的4个类别进行分类测试，以评估本体是否能有效支持文献分类应用，并探索在何种情况下本体能够最大限度支持分类。4个类别分别是治疗、风险因素、发病机制和康复。在评估过程中，采用6种不同方法进行对照：聚类、纯本体、深度学习模型、深度学习模型联合本体、大模型ChatGPT 3.5和大模型ChatGPT 4.0。在聚类方法中，使用K-means算法进行分

动脉粥样硬化性脑血管病本体构建与知识组织

Summary   Classes   Properties   Notes   Mappings   Widgets

Jump to:

- Clinical Manifestation
- Comorbidity
- Complication
- Diagnosis
  - Biomarkers in the diagnosis of Ath
    - Electrophysiological biomarkers c
    - Histological biomarkers of stroke
    - Molecular biomarkers of stroke
      - Apoptosis pathway markers
        - **B-type natriuretic peptide**
        - Beta globin DNA
        - N terminal proBNP
        - Nucleosomes
    - Glia biomarkers of stroke
    - Hemostatic biomarkers of strok
    - Inflammatory biomarkers of str
    - Neuronal biomarkers of stroke
    - Nonspecific markers of stroke
    - Oxidative stress biomarkers of s
    - Tissue destruction markers of s
    - Neuroimaging biomarkers of stro
    - OMICS biomarkers of stroke
    - Physical biomarkers of stroke
  - Brain anatomy
  - Differential diagnosis
  - Evaluation of Atherosclerotic Cereb
  - Pathway
- Model of Atherosclerotic Cerebrova
- pathogenesis
- Prevention
- Rehabilitation
- Risk factor
- Treatment

Details	Visualization Notes (0) Class Mappings (3)
Preferred Name	B-type natriuretic peptide
Synonyms	
ID	http://www.ustb.edu.cn/thesauri/tocr/v1/data#C571347974240595982
rdfs comment	Biomarker of Cardioembolic Stroke
altLabel	脑内素 脑钠肽 Brain natriuretic peptide 重组人脑利钠肽 BNP 血浆脑钠肽
dc source	http://purl.bioontology.org/ontology/MESH/D020097
definition	A PEPTIDE that is secreted by the BRAIN and the HEART ATRIA, stored mainly in cardiac ventricular MYOCARDIUM. It can cause NATRIURESIS, DIURESIS, VASODILATION, and inhibits secretion of RENIN and ALDOSTERONE. It improves heart function. It contains 32 AMINO ACIDS.
label	B型脑钠肽 B-type natriuretic peptide
oboInOwl:hasDbXref	http://purl.bioontology.org/ontology/SNOMEDCT/407059007 http://purl.bioontology.org/ontology/MESH/D020097
prefLabel	B-type natriuretic peptide
subClassOf	Apoptosis pathway markers

图1　本体术语展示界面

类。在纯本体方法中，使用抽取出的术语在本体中对应的概念及其所属类别来进行分类。在深度学习模型方法中，采用针对医学文献效果较好的PubmedBert模型进行分类预测。在深度学习模型联合本体的方法中，同样采用PubmedBert模型联合本体进行训练及预测。为此，课题组标注了600篇文献的所属分类，并对其进行划分，按照约为7∶3的比例进行训练集、测试集的划分。根据标注结果，对以上所有方法的P值（Precision）、R值（Recall）、$F1$值进行计算。公式如下，结果见表3，其中，样本量为n，属于分类i的样本量为$Count_i$，对应分类i的准确率P值、召回率R值和$F1$值分别是P_i、R_i、$F1_i$，对应加权P、R、$F1$值分别是$weight$-$P/R/F1$。

$$weighted\text{-}P = \sum_{i \in 1...n} W_i * P_i$$

$$weighted\text{-}R = \sum_{i \in 1...n} W_i * R_i$$

$$weighted\text{-}F1 = \sum_{i \in 1...n} W_i * F1_i$$

$$W_i = \frac{Count_i}{\sum_{i \in 1...n} Count_i}$$

表3　文本分类评估结果

算法	加权P值	加权R值	加权F1值
聚类（K-means）	62.32	40.40	45.18
纯本体	57.00	57.62	55.91
大模型GPT-3.5	76.60	66.23	68.23
大模型GPT-4.0	76.49	66.23	68.41
深度学习模型（PubMedBerT模型）	81.74	78.15	79.19
深度学习模型联合本体（Pub-MedBerT模型联合本体）	82.52	79.47	80.30

与聚类方法相比，使用纯本体进行简单分类的加权F1指标高出约24%，可以证明本体内容的准确度较高，能够支持文献分类的场景。与仅使用大模型的方法相比，可以最直观地体现本体的有效性。而联合本体预训练模型的分类效果达到80%，分类性能明显优于大模型GPT-3.5和GPT-4.0，表明该方法可能是对本体较为合理的利用方式。除文献分类外，仍有大量场景本体可以提供支持，以下内容为本体的部分扩展应用。

第二节　扩展应用

一、命名实体识别

本体包含动脉粥样硬化性脑血管病的相关概念，涵盖了该领域丰富的双语同义词，有助于实现自动标注与命名实体识别。课题组将本体导入到跨语言医学文本标注平台Comma（https://comma.phoc.org.cn/）中作为嵌入式词典，以供用户随时使用，而无须将本体定制为一个按要求格式上传的词典。自动标注的结果可以支持后续的数据训练和语料库的生成，还可大幅减少数据标注的成本和时间。同时，由于本体自身的清晰合理的知识体系结构，本体自动标注的命名实体识别将在很大程度上协助医生进行表型识别、诊断检查、治疗检索和效果识别，从而支持临床决策。

二、跨语言检索

本体可以通过扩展概念和范围自动辅助文献检索。面向特定领域的本体可以帮助文献检索实现更精确的文献或数据识别，例如，儿童疫苗接种本体对社会数据检索、收集和分析非常有用，有助于识别接种疫苗的儿童的情绪。再如，基于本体的护理知识平台可以进行信息检索和查询，提供相关知识的参考，更好地服务于护理。由于对动脉粥样硬化性脑血管病的认识尚未形成共识，这一领域的医生、医学信息学专家和研究人员需要对更多的知识和前沿成果，特别是医学文献进行深入研究。不同语言信息资源的不平衡可能导致知识分布的差异，因此，医生的跨语言需求不容忽视。不同国家的专家应有实现跨语言检索的途径。跨语言本体直接支持搜索策略的扩展和识别，在跨语言检索和综合搜索结果方面都具有独特的竞争力。

三、知识融合

现实世界的电子病历会产生大量的新术语或新表达。发现新术语，将新术语纳入原有知识体系，并恰当地融合到最适合的知识体系中具有重要意义。以上需求都可以借助当前本体来实现。在发现新术语的场景中，基于当前本体，可以通过命名实体识别算法对病历中的实体进行识别，通过规则和相似度检测算法进行候选术语筛选，完成新的表达检测，并最终实现新术语的确定。而在获得新术语之后，同样可以基于原有本体与新术语的相似度匹配算法实现新术语的待融合实体匹配，并完成对新术语的最终融合，扩展本体，不断形成知识粒度更细，知识内容更丰富，合理的、有价值的知识体系。

第四章

结　语

　　动脉粥样硬化性脑血管病作为一种高发且危害性极高的疾病，一直没有得到足够的重视。截至目前，其尚未获得学术界的共识，因此没有已发布的系统的概念数据集来帮助该领域的临床医生明确范围和辅助研究。当前本体旨在解决上述科学问题，提供一套清晰的跨语言概念和术语，具有明确的层次结构，能帮助科研人员快速检索相关医学文献，帮助数据科学家高效识别电子健康记录等医学数据中的相关内容，并提供清晰的领域框架供学术参考。本体当前还不够全面，无法包含该领域发生的所有信息，需要时时更新。例如，随着康复设备的不断升级，及时扩充与更新康复术语，并提供更丰富与精准的检索、实体识别、支持文献分类等功能。在未来的工作中，我们会不断完善动脉粥样硬化性脑血管病涉及的内容，并最大程度辅助临床诊疗。课题组将对动脉粥样硬化性脑血管病数据集进行公开发布以支持领域科研人员进行利用与研究。

参 考 文 献

［1］TSANTILAS P, LAO S, WU Z, et al. Chitinase 3 like 1 is a regulator of smooth muscle cell physiology and atherosclerotic lesion stability［J］. Cardiovasc Res, 2021, 117(14): 2767-2780.

［2］LEE S C, SON K J, HOON HAN C, et al. Cardiovascular and cerebrovascular-associated mortality in patients with preceding bronchiectasis exacerbation［J］. Ther Adv Respir Dis, 2022, 16: 17534666221144206.

［3］HERON M. Deaths: leading causes for 2019［J］. Natl Vital Stat Rep, 2021, 70(9): 1-114.

［4］DONNAN G A, FISHER M, MACLEOD M, et al. Stroke［J］. Lancet, 2008, 371(9624): 1612-1623.

［5］SAINI V, GUADA L, YAVAGAL D R. Global epidemiology of stroke and access to acute ischemic stroke interventions［J］. Neurology, 2021, 97(20 Suppl 2): S6-S16.

［6］VIRANI S S, ALONSO A, BENJAMIN E J, et al. Heart disease and stroke statistics-2020 update: a report from the American Heart Association［J］. Circulation, 2020, 141(9): e139-e596.

［7］BARTHELS D, DAS H. Current advances in ischemic stroke research and therapies［J］. Biochim Biophys Acta Mol Basis Dis, 2020, 1866(4): 165260.

［8］KHOSHNAM S E, WINLOW W, FARZANEH M, et al. Pathogenic mechanisms following ischemic stroke［J］. Neurol Sci, 2017, 38(7): 1167-1186.

［9］TSUCHIYA M, SAKO K, YURA S, et al. Cerebral blood flow and histopathological changes following permanent bilateral carotid artery ligation in Wistar rats［J］. Exp Brain Res, 1992, 89(1): 87-92.

［10］GBD 2016 Stroke Collaborators. Global, regional, and national burden of stroke, 1990-2016: a systematic analysis for the Global Burden of Disease Study 2016［J］. Lancet Neurol, 2019, 18(5): 439-458.

［11］SAFAROVA M S, KULLO I J. Using the electronic health record for genomics research［J］. Curr Opin Lipidol, 2020, 31(2): 85-93.

［12］章成国. 动脉粥样硬化性血管疾病［M］. 北京: 人民卫生出版社, 2015.

［13］LIU L, CHEN W, ZHOU H, et al. Chinese Stroke Association guidelines for clinical management of cerebrovascular disorders: executive summary and 2019 update of clinical management of ischaemic cerebrovascular diseases［J］. Stroke Vasc Neurol, 2020, 5(2): 159-176.

［14］WANG J, BAI L, SHI M, et al. Trends in age of first-ever stroke following increased incidence and life expectancy in a low-income Chinese population［J］. Stroke, 2016, 47(4): 929-935.

［15］MOZAFFARIAN D, BENJAMIN E J, GO A S, et al. Heart disease and stroke statistics—2015 update: a report from the American Heart Association［J］. Circulation, 2015, 131(4):

e29-e322.

［16］WINSTEIN C J, STEIN J, ARENA R, et al. Guidelines for adult stroke rehabilitation and re-covery: a guideline for healthcare professionals from the American Heart Association/American Stroke Association［J］. Stroke, 2016, 47(6): e98-e169.

［17］BUNTIN M B, COLLA C H, DEB P, et al. Medicare spending and outcomes after postacute care for stroke and hip fracture［J］. Med Care, 2010, 48(9): 776-784.

［18］SAINI V, GUADAL, YAVAGALDR. 2021. Global Bpidemiology of stroke and access to acute ischemic stroke interventions. Neurology, 97, S6-S16.

［19］ORNELLO R, DEGAN D, TISEO C, et al. Distribution and temporal trends from 1993 to 2015 of ischemic stroke subtypes: a systematic review and meta-analysis［J］. Stroke, 2018, 49(4): 814-819.

［20］KOH S H, PARK H H. Neurogenesis in stroke recovery［J］. Transl Stroke Res, 2017, 8(1): 3-13.

［21］CRAMER S C, CHOPP M. Recovery recapitulates ontogeny［J］. Trends Neurosci, 2000, 23(6): 265-271.

［22］National Institute of Neurological Disorders and Stroke rt-PA Stroke Study Group. Tissue plas-minogen activator for acute ischemic stroke［J］. N Engl J Med, 1995, 333(24): 1581-1587.

［23］HABIBI-KOOLAEE M, SHAHMORADI L, NIAKAN KALHORI S R, et al. STO: stroke on-tology for accelerating translational stroke research［J］. Neurol Ther, 2021, 10(1): 321-333.

［24］KÖHLER S, GARGANO M, MATENTZOGLU N, et al. The Human Phenotype Ontology in 2021［J］. Nucleic Acids Res, 2021, 49(D1): D1207-D1217.

［25］NOY N F, MCGUINNESS D L. Ontology development 101: a guide to creating your first ontology［C］. 2001. http: //protege. stanford. edu/publications/ontology. development/ontolo-gylol. pdf.

附录A

动脉粥样硬化性脑血管病术语集

英文术语	中文术语
10 - Dysarthria	10-构音障碍
11 - Extinction and Inattention	11-消失和注意力不集中
1a - Level of Consciousness	1a - 意识水平
1b - Level of Consciousness Questions	1b-意识水平提问
1c - Level of Consciousness Commands	1c-意识水平指令
2 - Best Gaze	2-凝视
3 - Visual	3 - 视野
3-nitrotyrosine; 3 nitrotyrosine	3-硝基酪氨酸
4 - Facial Palsy	4—面瘫
5a - Motor Arm - right	5a-右臂运动
5b - Motor Arm - left	5b-左臂运动
6a - Motor Leg - right	6a-右腿运动
6b - Motor Leg - left	6b-左腿运动
7 - Limb Ataxia	7-肢体共济失调
8 - Sensory	8-感觉
8-hydroxy-2-deoxy-guanosine; 8 hydroxy 2 deoxy guanosine	8-羟基-2-脱氧鸟苷
9 - Best Language	9-最佳语言
Abasia	行走不稳
abciximab	阿昔单抗
ABCs; Airway breathing circulation control	复苏抢救ABC；气道呼吸循环控制
Abdominal obesity; Central obesity; central obesity; Truncal obesity; Centripetal obesity; Central obesity (disorder)	腹型肥胖；向心性肥胖；躯干性肥胖；中心性肥胖
Abduction palsy; Outward paralysis	外展神经麻痹；外展性瘫痪
Abnormal Amsler grid test	阿姆斯勒方格表检查异常
Abnormal automated kinetic perimetry test	自动动态视野检查异常

续　表

英文术语	中文术语
Abnormal confrontational visual field test; Abnormal face-to-face visual field test; Abnormal confrontational visual field examination; Abnormal face-to-face visual field examination	异常对抗视野测试；面对面视野检查异常
Abnormal Estermann grid perimetry test	Estermann 网格视野检查异常
Abnormal fibrinolytic system; Abnormal fibrinolysis system; Abnormal coagulation system; Abnormal plasminogen system	纤溶系统异常
Abnormal Humphrey SITA 10-2 perimetry test	Humphrey SITA 10-2 视野检查异常
Abnormal Humphrey SITA 24-2 perimetry test	Humphrey SITA 24-2 视野检查异常
Abnormal Humphrey SITA 30-2 perimetry test	Humphrey SITA 30-2 视野检查异常
Abnormal kinetic perimetry test	动态视野检查异常
Abnormal manual kinetic perimetry test	手工动态视野检查异常
Abnormal plasminogen; Plasminogen abnormality; Plasminogen aberrant; Plasminogen disorder	纤溶酶原异常
Abnormal static automated perimetry test	自动静态视野检查异常
Abnormal static perimetry test	静态视野检查异常
Abnormal visual field test; Abnormal visual field examination; aberrant visual field examination; anomaly visual field examination	视野检查异常；异常视野检查
Acalculia; acalculia; Acalculia (finding)	失算；失算症
Acetyl polyamine oxidase; AcPAO	乙酰基聚胺氧化酶
Acrolein	丙烯醛；丙烯腈；丙烯酸
Action tremor; action tremor; kinetic tremor	动作性震颤；活动性震颤
Activated protein C; APC	活化蛋白C
Activation of sigma receptors; Activation of sigma receptor; Sigma receptors activation; Sigma receptor activation	σ受体激活；激活σ受体
active exercise; active movement; active motions; initiative movement; active movement treatment; active movement ability; early active movement; active locomotion	主动运动；主动训练；主动锻炼法；主动运动训练；主动锻炼；练习主动性；主动活动
Active protein C resistance Leiden type; activated protein c resistance	活性蛋白C抗性莱顿型；活性蛋白C耐药莱顿型
active-operative EMG-BF; Active-operational electromechanical biofeedback	主动性(操作性)肌电生物反馈疗法；肌电生物反馈疗法

续　表

英文术语	中文术语
activities of daily life abilities; activities of daily living; basic activities of daily living; Actibities of Daily Living; basic activity of daily living	日常生活能力；基础性日常生活能力
Acupuncture; acupuncture-moxibustion; acupuncture therapy; needle moxibustion; acupuncture treatment; acupunture; Manual acupuncture; moxi-acupuncture; acupuncture and moxibustion	针灸；针刺疗法；针灸疗法；针刺治疗；针灸学；针灸治疗；针术；针刺术
Acute agitated delirium; Acute agitation delirium	急性躁狂性谵妄；急性激动性谵妄
Acute confusional state	急性意识模糊状态；急性精神混乱状态；急性意识模糊发作
Acute hypertension; Acute high blood pressure	急性高血压；高血压急症；急性高血压性；急症高血压
Acute necrotizing encephalopathy	急性坏死性脑病
Acute unilateral deafness; Acute unilateral hearing loss	急性单侧耳聋；急性一侧耳聋
adenosine; Increase of adenosine	腺苷；腺苷增加；腺甙；腺嘌呤核苷；腺苷脱氨酶；腺苷酸；阿糖腺苷；腺苷虫
Adenosine diphosphate; ADP	二磷酸腺苷；腺嘌呤核苷二磷酸；多聚二磷酸腺苷；腺苷二磷酸(ADP)；腺苷二磷酸；二磷腺苷；腺嘌呤核甙二磷酸；二磷酸腺甙
Adiponectin; Leptin; Adipsin	脂联素；脂联素基因；脂连素；脂连蛋白
Adjusted clinical group; ACGs; ACG	调整临床组
Adult polycystic kidney disease; adult polycystic kidney	成人型多囊肾病；成人多囊肾病
Adynamic aphasia; unpowered aphasia	丧动力性失语；动态失语症；动力缺失失语症
aerobic exercise; Aerobic physical activity; aerobic endurance training	有氧运动；趣味性有氧运动
Aerodynamics check; Gas dynamics inspection	气体动力学检查；气动力学检查；空气动力学检查
Afibrinogenemia; afibrinogenemia; Afibrinogenaemia; Afibrinogenemia (disorder)	纤维蛋白原缺乏血症
Age factor; Age factors; Older age	年龄因素；年龄

续　表

英文术语	中文术语
Agraphia; agraphia; Agraphia (finding)	失写；失写症
Akathisia; akathisia; Agitation confusional state; Agitated confusional state; Akithisia; Akathisia (disorder)	静坐不能；失静症；静坐失能
Akinetic mutism; Akinetic autism; Akinetic mutism (disorder); Mutism; Muteness; akinetic mutism	无动性缄默；缄默症；运动不能性缄默；运动不能性缄默症；运动不能缄默症
Albert Test; Albert's Test	艾伯特测试；Albert测试
Alberta stroke program early CT score; ASPECTS	艾伯塔中风计划早期CT评分；Alberta中风计划早期CT评分
Alcohol drinking; Alcohol consumption; Alcohol intake; consumption of alcohol	饮酒；饮酒行为；饮酒情况；嗜酒者；饮酒量；乙醇摄入
Alexia with agraphia; Aphasia with Miswriting; dyslexia with Miswriting	失读症伴失写；失读症伴绘画不能；失读症伴书写不能
Alexia without agraphia syndrome; pure alexia; letter-by-letter dyslexia; pure word blindness; agnosic alexia	失读不伴失写综合征；失读无失写综合征
alpha 2 macroglobulin; alpha-2-macroglobulin; a-2-macroglobulin	α2巨球蛋白
alpha blockers; α-blocker	α受体阻滞剂；α阻滞剂
alpha phenyl 2 pyridineethanamine dihydrochloride; AR-R15896AR	α苯基2吡啶乙胺二盐酸盐
Alpha tocopherol; Alpha-tocopherol; a-tocopherol	维生素E；α-生育酚
Altitudinal visual field defect; Vertical visual field defect; perpendicular visual field defect	垂直视野缺损
Amaurosis fugax; amaurosis fugax; AMAUROSIS FUGAX; AF - Amaurosis fugax; AFx - Amaurosis fugax; Amaurosis fugax (one sided temporary vision loss); Amaurosis fugax (disorder)	一过性黑矇；短暂性失明；一时性黑蒙；一时性黑矇；一过性黑朦；暂时性黑朦
American Speech & Hearing Association Functional Assesement of Communication Skills; ASHA-FACS	美国言语与听力学会交流能力功能性评价
Amnesia; amnesia; Amnestic disorder; Amnestic syndrome; Amnesic syndrome; Amnestic disorder (disorder)	健忘症；健忘；遗忘症；器质性遗忘综合征；遗忘综合症；遗忘-虚构综合征；Korsakoff综合征；柯萨可夫病；遗忘障碍；柯萨可夫综合征；遗忘综合征
Amphetamine; amphetamine; Amfetamine	安非他明；苯丙胺

续　表

英文术语	中文术语
Amsterdam Nijmegen Everyday Language Test; ANELT	Amsterdam Nijmegen 日常语言测试
Amusia; amusia; Amusia (finding)	失音症；失乐感
Amyloid plaques	淀粉样蛋白斑；淀粉样斑；淀粉斑；淀粉样斑块
Anacetrapib	安塞曲比
Anarthria; Jumbled speech; Anarthria (finding)	构音障碍；音节不清；口吃
Ancrod	安克洛酶；蛇毒去纤维酶；蛇毒蛋白酶；去纤维酶类
Anemia; Anemias; Haemolytic anaemias; haemolytic anemia; hemolytic anemia; Hemolytic anemia; anemia; Anaemia; anaemia; Haemolytic anaemia; Hemolytic anemia (disorder); Absolute anemia; Absolute anaemia; Anemia (disorder); Anaemia (disorder)	贫血；溶血性贫血；绝对性贫血
Aneurysm recurrence; recurrent aneurysm	动脉瘤复发
Angiogenesis; tumor angiogenesis; neovascularization; vascularization; angiogenesis growth; angiogenic; vascular formation; blood vessels' formation	血管生成；血管新生；血管形成；肿瘤血管生成；血管发生；新生血管生成；血管化；血管增生
Angioplasty; Endovascular angioplasty and stenting; Angioplasty and stenting; Balloon angioplasty	血管成形术；血管成型术；冠脉成形术；腔内成形术；血管再造；血管成形
angiopoietin 2; ANGPT2	血管生成素2
angiopoietin signaling pathway; angiogenin signaling pathway; angiopoietins signaling pathway	血管生成素信号通路
angiotensin converting enzyme inhibitors; ACE inhibitors; ACEI; angiotensin converting enzyme inhibition; angiotensin-converting inhibitors; angiotensin-converting inhibition; angiotensin receptor blockers; angiotensin-converting enzyme inhibiter	血管紧张素转化酶抑制剂；血管紧张素转换酶抑制药；血管转换酶抑制剂；血管紧张肽转化酶抑制药；血管紧张素转化抑制剂
angiotensin I-converting enzyme; ACE DD genotype; ACE; angiotonin I convertase	血管紧张素转换酶；血管紧张素I转换酶基因；血管紧张素 I 转化酶；血管紧张素I转化酶
Anisocoria; anisocoria; Asymmetry of the pupils; Asymmetric pupil sizes; Unequal pupil size; Unequal pupils; Anisocoria (disorder)	瞳孔不等；瞳孔不等大；瞳孔不均
Anistreplase	阿尼普酶
Ankle-foot Orthosis; AFOs	踝足矫形器；踝足支架

续　表

英文术语	中文术语
Anomalous trichromacy; Trichromatic anomalies	三色视觉障碍；异常三色视
Anosodiaphoria; Anosodiaphoria (finding)	疾病淡漠
Anosognosia; anosognosia; Anosognosia (finding)	疾病失认症；病感失认症；病感失认
Anterior cerebral artery; anterior cerebral artery; Anterior cerebral arteries; ACAs; ACA	大脑前动脉
Anterior cerebral artery infarction syndrome; syndromes of anterior cerebral artery infarction; syndrome of anterior cerebral artery infarction; Anterior cerebral artery infarction syndromes; Anterior cerebral artery infarction symptoms; Anterior cerebral artery infarction symptom; ACA infarction symptom	大脑前动脉梗死综合征
Anterior choroidal artery; Anterior choroidal arteries; AChAs; AChA	前脉络丛动脉
Anterior choroidal artery infarction syndrome; syndromes of anterior choroidal artery infarction; syndrome of anterior choroidal artery infarction; Anterior choroidal artery infarction syndromes; Anterior choroidal artery infarction symptoms; Anterior choroidal artery infarction symptom; AChA infarction symptom; Syndromes of Anterior Choroidal Artery Territory Infarction	脉络膜前动脉梗死综合征
Anterior communicating artery; Anterior communicating arteries; ACoAs; ACoA; anterior communicating artery	前交通动脉
Anterior inferior cerebellar artery; Anterior inferior cerebellar arteries; AICAs; AICA	小脑前下动脉
Anterior inferior cerebellar artery embolism; anterior inferior cerebellar artery embolism; anterior inferior cerebellum embolism; Anterior inferior cerebellar artery embolization; Anterior inferior cerebellar artery thromboembolism	小脑前下动脉栓塞；小脑前下动脉血栓栓塞
Anterior inferior cerebellar artery infarction symptom; AICA infarction symptom	小脑前下动脉梗死症状；小脑前下动脉梗塞症状
Anterograde amnesia; Antegrade amnesia; Anterograde amnesia (finding); anterograde amnesia	顺行性遗忘；顺行健忘症；顺行性遗忘症
anticoagulants; Anticoagulation drugs therapy; Anticoagulation agents; Anticoagulation drugs; Anticoagulation agent; Anticoagulation drug; Anticoagulants; Anticoagulant; anticoagulant	抗凝剂；抗凝血剂；抗凝血药
Antiedema Therapy; Medical Antiedema Therapy	降颅压；抗水肿疗法；抗水肿治疗

续　表

英文术语	中文术语
Antihyperlipidemic agents; Lipid lowering therapies; Lipid-modifying therapy; Lipid lowering therapy; Lipid-lowering agents; lipid lowering drugs; Hypolipidemic agents; Lipid-lowering agent; lipid-lowering drugs; lipid-lowering drug; lipid lowering drug; Treating high blood lipid level; Cholesterol lowering therapies; Cholesterol lowering therapy	调脂药物；降血脂药物；降血脂药
Antihypertensive drugs therapy; Blood pressure medications; vasopressor drugs therapy; Blood pressure medication	降压药物治疗；抗高血压药物治疗
Antileukocytic antibody; human antileukocytic antibody	破坏白细胞的抗体
Antioxidants; antioxidant; antioxidants; antioxygen; antioxidant agent; antioxidant activity	抗氧化剂；抗氧剂；抗氧化；抗氧化药；抗氧化物；抗氧化性；抗氧化酶
Antiphospholipid syndrome; Antiphospholipid antibody syndrome; APAS; APS; antiphospholipid syndrome; APL - Antiphospholipid syndrome; APS - Antiphospholipid syndrome; Anticardiolipin syndrome; Antiphospholipid syndrome (disorder)	抗磷脂抗体综合征；抗磷脂综合征；抗心磷脂抗体综合征；抗磷脂综合症；抗磷脂抗体综合症
Antiplatelet antibodies; anti-platelet antibodies; antiplatelet antibody; platelet antibody; platelet associated immunoglobulin	抗血小板抗体
Antiplatelet drugs; Antiplatelet drugs therapy; Antithrombotic treatment; Antithrombotic therapy; Platelet antagonists; Antiplatelet therapy; Platelet antagonist; Antiplatelet agents; Thromboprophylactic; Thromboprophylaxis; Antiplatelet agent; Antiplatelet drug	抗血小板药物治疗；抗血小板药物疗法
Aortic atherosclerosis; Atherosclerosis of aorta; aortic atherosclerosis; abdominal aortosclerosis; Atherosclerosis of aorta (disorder); Atherosclerosis aorta; Abdominal aortic atherosclerosis; Atherosclerosis of abdominal aorta; Abdominal aortic atherosclerosis (disorder)	主动脉动脉粥样硬化；主动脉粥样硬化；主动脉硬化；主动脉粥样硬化症；腹主动脉粥样硬化
Apathy; apathy; abulia; Indifference; Abulia; Indifferent mood; Emotionally apathetic; Indifference (finding)	淡漠；意志丧失；意志缺失；意志力丧失；情感淡漠
Aphasic Depression Rating Scale; ADRS	失语抑郁量表
Apixaban	阿哌沙班

英文术语	中文术语
Aplastic anemia; Aplastic Anemias; Aplastic anaemia; aplastic anaemia; aplastic anemia; Regenerative anemia; Hypoproliferative anemia; Hypoproliferative anaemia; Regenerative anaemia; Anaemia with regeneration; Anemia with regeneration; Aplastic anemia (disorder)	再生障碍性贫血；低增殖性贫血；再生性贫血；再生障碍性贫血(AA)
APOE	载脂蛋白 E
APOH; Apolipoprotein H	载脂蛋白 H
Apolipoprotein A-I; ApoA1; ApoA 1; Apo AI; Apo-AI; ApoA-1	载脂蛋白 A-I
Apolipoprotein B; Apo-B; Apo B; ApoB	载脂蛋白 B
Apolipoprotein C1; Apo CI; Apo C1	载脂蛋白 C1
Apolipoprotein C3; Apo CIII; Apo C3	载脂蛋白 C3
Apolipoprotein E epsilon 2 allele; apoE epsilon 2 allele	载脂蛋白 Eε2 等位基因
Apoptosis; Gene-directed cell death; Programmed cell death; PCD	细胞凋亡；基因导向的细胞死亡；细胞程序性死亡
Apoptosis inducing factor; apoptosis induced factor; apoptosis induce factor; apoptosis factor; apoptosis-including factor; apoptosis inducing factor protein; AIF	凋亡诱导因子；凋亡因子
Apoptosis pathway markers; Apoptosis pathway marker	凋亡途径标志物
apoptotic cell death pathway; programmed cell death pathway; Pathway of apoptosis cell death	凋亡细胞死亡途径
Apraxia; apraxia; Apraxia (finding)	失用症；失用
Arcuate scotoma; arcuate scotoma; Arcuate defects; Arcuate scotoma (finding)	弧形暗点；弓形暗点；弓形盲点缺损；弓形盲点
Arginase 1; ARG1	精氨酸酶 1
Arnadottir OT ADL Neurobehavioral Evaluation; A-ONE	Arnadottir OT ADL 神经行为评估
Arterial circulation	动脉循环
Arterial embolism; arterial embolism; Arterial thrombosis; Arterial thrombosis (disorder); Arterial embolus; Arterial embolism, NOS, of unspecified artery; Arterial embolism (disorder)	动脉栓塞；动脉栓塞症；急性动脉栓塞；动脉血栓栓塞；动脉栓塞形成
Arterial Hypertension; Arterial high blood pressure	动脉性高血压；动脉高压；动脉高血压的；动脉高血压；原发性高血压
Arterial Hypotension	低动脉压；动脉压过低

续　表

英文术语	中文术语
Artery-to-artery embolism; Interarterial embolization; Artery to artery embolism; Arteriogenic embolism	动脉-动脉栓塞；动脉栓塞
ASCO Phenotypic System; atherosclerosis, small vessel disease, cardiac source, and other cause; ASCO	Asco表型系统
Ascorbic acid; Vitamin C; ascorbic acid; vitamin C	维生素C；抗坏血酸
Asomatognosia; Asomatognosia (finding); Disturbance of body schema	躯体失认症；自体感觉缺失
aspartate; Increase of aspartate	天冬胺酰胺；天冬氨酸盐；天冬氨酸增加；天冬氨酸根；天冬氨酸酯；天冬氨酸
Aspirin; Aspirin therapy; ASA; aspirin	阿司匹林；阿斯匹林；阿司匹林肠溶片
assessment of cognitive function; cognitive assessment; cognition assessment; cognitive function assessment	认知功能评估；认知功能评分；认知功能评定
Assessment of Motor and Process Skills; AMPS	运动和过程技能评估
Astasia; Thalamic astasia	站立不能；起立不能
Asterixis; asterixis; ASTERIXIS; Flapping tremor; Asterixis (finding)	扑翼样震颤；姿势保持不能；扑动状震颤；扑翼性震颤
Astrocyte; cultured astrocytes; astrocyte cell; cortical astrocytes; astroglial cell; glial cells; astrocyte cells; Astrocytes	星形胶质细胞；星形细胞
Asynergia; asynergia; Asynergia (finding)	共济失调；协同动作不能；协同不能；协调不能
Ataxic hemiparesis; Ataxic hemiparesis syndrome; Crural paresis; Ataxic hemiparesis (disorder)	震颤性轻偏瘫；抽搐性偏瘫
Atherosclerotic Cerebrovascular Disease team; Atherosclerotic Cerebrovascular Disease group	动脉粥样硬化性脑血管病小组
Atorvastatin	阿托伐他汀；阿托伐他汀钙；阿托伐他；瑞舒伐他汀；阿托伐他丁
ATP depletion	ATP耗竭；ATP损耗；ATP缺失；ATP骤降；ATP含量下降
Atrial arrhythmia; atrial arrhythmia; Atrial arrhythmia (disorder)	房性心律失常；房性心律不齐
Atrial fibrillation; atrial fibrillation; AF - Atrial fibrillation; Atrial fibrillation (disorder); AF	心房颤动；心房纤颤；房颤；心房颤动(心房纤颤)；房性纤颤

续　表

英文术语	中文术语
Atrial natriuretic factor; ANF	心房利钠因子；心房钠尿因子；心房利纳肽因子
attention; mental concentration; attention ability; attention economy; concentration; attention mechanism; attentiveness	注意力；注意；关注度；关注
Auditory agnosia; auditory agnosia; Acoustic agnosia; Auditory agnosia (finding)	听觉失认；听觉失认症
Auditory hallucinations; auditory hallucination; acoasma; Auditory Hallucinations; Auditory hallucination; Auditory hallucinations (finding)	幻听
augmentative and alternative communication system; Enhanced alternating communication facilitation therapy; AAC	增强交替交流促进疗法
Automatic voluntary dissociation with facial paresis; Automatic voluntary dissociation with facial paresis，Automatic voluntary separation with facial palsy	自动分离性面部轻瘫；自动自愿性分离伴面瘫
Axial dystonia	轴向肌张力障碍
B type neurotrophic growth factor; B-type neurotrophic growth factor	B 型神经营养生长因子
B-type natriuretic peptide; Brain natriuretic peptide; BNP	B 型脑钠肽；脑钠素；重组人脑利钠肽；血浆脑钠肽；脑钠肽
balance function; equilibrium function; balance funtion; balancing function; balance disability; balance ability	平衡功能；平衡机能；平衡能力
Balint syndrome; Cortical paralysis of fixation syndrome; Cortical paralysis of fixation syndrome (disorder); Balint's syndrome	巴林特综合征；凝视性皮质麻痹综合征；皮层性注视麻痹；Balint 综合征；Holmes-Horrax 综合征；皮质性注视麻痹综合征；视固定皮质性麻痹综合征
Barbiturate	巴比妥盐；巴比妥酸盐；巴比妥酸
Barthel Index; BI	Barthel 指数
Basal ganglia; basal nucleus; basal ganglion; basal ganglion areas	基底节；基底核；基底神经结；基底神经节
Basilar artery; Basilar arteries; BAs; BA; basilar artery	基底动脉
Basilar artery atherosclerosis; Basal artery atherosclerotic plaque; basilar artery plaque; basilar artery atherosclerosis; basilar atherosclerosis; symptomatic basilar artery atherosclerosis	基底动脉粥样硬化；基底动脉粥样硬化斑块形成

续　表

英文术语	中文术语
Basilar artery infarction syndrome; syndromes of basilar artery infarction; syndrome of basilar artery infarction; Basilar artery infarction syndromes; Basilar artery infarction symptoms; Basilar artery infarction symptom; BA infarction symptom	基底动脉梗死综合征
bathing; bath; wash; tub; take a shower; bathe; shower taking	洗澡；沐浴
Beck Depression Inventory Ⅱ	贝克抑郁量表Ⅱ；Beck 抑郁自评问卷Ⅱ；Beck 抑郁自评量表 Ⅱ
Bedside seat retention; Bedside seat keeping	床边坐位保持
Behavior compensation strategy; compensatory strategy; Compensatory strategy	行为补偿；代偿性策略；补偿性策略；行为补偿法
Behavioral disturbance; behaviour disorder; abnormal behaviour; behavioral abnormality; behavioral disorders; behavior disorder	行为异常；行为障碍
Behavioral Inattention Test; BIT	行为学忽略测试
Bell's palsy; Lower motor neuron facial nerve palsy; Bell palsy; Bells palsy; Bell's palsy (disorder)	Bell 麻痹；贝尔氏麻痹；贝尔面瘫；贝耳氏麻痹；贝尔麻痹；贝尔麻痹(面神经麻痹)；周围性面瘫
Benedikt syndrome; benedikt syndrome; Benedikt's syndrome; Tegmentum syndrome; Benedict syndrome; Benedikt's syndrome (disorder); Mesencephalic tegmental paralysis; paramedian midbrain syndrome	Benedikt 综合征；贝内迪克特综合征；贝内迪克特综合征(一侧动眼神经麻痹、对侧肢体轻瘫及震颤)；本尼迪特氏综合征(一侧动眼神经瘫痪)；Benedict 综合征
Berg balance scale	Berg 平衡评价量表
beta blockers; beta-blocker; beta receptor blocker; beta-receptor blockers; beta-blocker therapy; beta-adrenergic blocker; adrenergic beta-antagonists	β受体阻滞剂；β受体阻断剂；β受体阻滞剂药
Beta carotene intake; Beta carotene supplements	β胡萝卜素摄入量
Beta globin DNA	β球蛋白 DNA；β珠蛋白 DNA
Beta thromboglobulin; b-thromboglobulin; PPBP	β凝血球蛋白
Betamethasone	倍他米松；培他米松；倍他美松 ；倍氟美松
Bilateral ptosis; double sides ptosis; Bilateral eyelid ptosis; two-sided ptosis	双侧上睑下垂；双侧眼睑下垂；两侧上睑下垂

续　表

英文术语	中文术语
Bilateral vision loss; bilateral decreased visual acuity; bilateral impaired vision; bilateral decreased vision; bilateral vision loss; bilateral visual acuity loss; bilateral decreased eyesight; bilateral visual impairment; bilateral vision decrease	双侧视力下降；双侧视力障碍；双侧视力损伤；双侧视力减退
Bilateral weakness; Bilateral incapacity	双侧无力；双边无力；两侧无力
Bile acid sequestrants; bile acid binding agent; Bile acid sequestrant antilipemic agen	胆酸结合剂；胆汁酸多价螯合剂
Binasal hemianopia; Binasal hemianopsia; Binasal hemianopia (finding); binasal hemianopsia	双鼻侧偏盲；鼻侧偏盲；双内侧偏盲；两鼻侧偏盲
Binswanger disease; Subcortical leucoencephalopathy; Binswanger's dementia; Binswanger's disease; Binswanger's encephalopathy; Subcortical arteriosclerotic encephalopathy; Subcortical atherosclerotic dementia; Subcortical leukoencephalopathy (disorder); Subcortical leukoencephalopathy; Binswanger's disease; BD; binswanger disease	皮层下白质脑病；皮质下动脉硬化性脑病；宾斯旺格(氏)病；皮层下动脉硬化性脑病；Binswanger病；宾斯万格病；动脉硬化性皮层下脑病；进行性皮层下血管性脑病；宾斯旺格氏病；宾斯万格氏病；进行性白质脑病；宾斯旺格病
biofeedback therapy; biological feedback therapy; EFT	生物反溃治疗；生物反馈疗法
Biomarkers in the diagnosis of Atherosclerotic Cerebrovascular Disease; Atherosclerotic Cerebrovascular Disease biomarkers; Atherosclerotic Cerebrovascular Disease biomarker	诊断动脉粥样硬化性脑血管病的生物标志物；动脉粥样硬化性脑血管病诊断中的生物标志物
Bitemporal hemianopia; bitemporal hemianopsia; Bitemporal hemianopsia; Bitemporal hemianopia (finding)	双颞侧偏盲；两颞侧偏盲；双外侧偏盲
Blepharospasm; blepharospasm; Spasm of eyelids; Essential blepharospasm; Benign essential blepharospasm; Blepharospasm (spasm of eyelid); Blepharospasm (disorder)	眼睑痉挛；睑痉挛
Blind-spot enlargment; Enlarged blind spot; physiological blind spot enlarged; Enlarged angioscotoma; Enlarged paracaecal scotoma; Enlarged blind spot (finding)	生理盲点扩大；盲点扩大
blood glucose test; Blood sugar test; blood glucose testing	血糖检验；血糖检测；血糖试验；血葡萄糖测定
Blood pressure; blood pressure; BP	血压；脉压
blood pressure biofeedback therapy; BPBFT	血压生物反馈疗法
Blood pressure control; hypertension control; blood pressure controlling; pressure control; hypertenion control	控制血压；血压控制；血压调控；血压调节

续　表

英文术语	中文术语
Bobath evaluation method	Bobath 评测法
Bobath neurodevelopmental treatment; Bobath neurodevelopmental therapy; Bobath neurodevelopment treatment; Bobath neural developmental approach	Bobath 神经发育疗法；Bobath法
Body temperature; temperature; thermoregulation	体温；体温度
bone mineral density measurement	骨密度测定；骨密度测量；骨矿物密度测定；骨密度检测
Boston Diagnostic Aphasia Examination; BDAE	波士顿诊断性失语症检查
Boston Naming Test	Boston 命名测验
Box and Block Test; BB test; BBT	箱块试验
Brain abscess; brain abscess; Abscess of brain; Cerebral abscess; BRAIN ABSCESS; Cerebral abscess (disorder); Abscess of brain (disorder)	脑脓肿；大脑脓肿；颅内脓肿；颅脑脓肿
brain derived neurotrophic factor; BDNF	脑源性神经营养因子
Brain imaging; neuroimage; brain image; brain imaging technique	脑成像；脑显像；脑显象；大脑成像；颅脑影像；脑功能成像
Brain region; cerebral areas; brain area; brain areas	脑部区域；脑分区；大脑分区
Brain tumor; Brain tumors; Intracranial tumors; Intracranial tumor; intracranial tumour; intracranial tumor; Intracranial tumour; Brain tumour; BT - Brain tumor; BT - Brain tumour; ICT - Intracranial tumor; ICT - Intracranial tumour; Intracranial neoplasm; Intracranial tumor (disorder)	脑肿瘤；颅内肿瘤；脑瘤；中枢神经系统肿瘤；颅脑肿瘤；BT-脑肿瘤；ICT-颅内肿瘤；BT - 脑肿瘤
Brain type fatty acid binding protein; B-FABP; BFABP	脑型脂肪酸结合蛋白
brain-derived neurotrophic factor signaling pathway; BDNF signaling pathway	脑源性神经营养因子信号通路
Brainstem; brainstem; brain stem; Brain Stem	脑桥；中脑
Brainstem infarct syndrome; syndromes of brainstem infarct; syndrome of brainstem infarct; Brainstem infarct syndromes; Brainstem infarct symptoms; Brainstem infarct symptom	脑干梗死综合征
Broca aphasia; Broca-type aphasia	Broca 失语；布罗卡失语症；布罗卡失语；布洛卡失语症；Broca 失语症

英文术语	中文术语
Broccoli; cauliflower; cauliflowers	花椰菜；硬花球花柳；青花椰菜；木立花椰莱；抽条的花茎甘蓝
brunnstrom	Brunnstrom评定法
Brunnstrom movement therapy; Brunnstrom exercise therapy; Brunnstrom kinesitherapy; Brunnstrom exercise treatment	Brunnstrom运动疗法；Brunnstrom法
Buccofacial apraxia; Orofacial apraxia	颊面失用症
Butter intake; Butter	黄油摄入量
Bypass surgery; bypass graft surgery; bypass grafting surgery; bypass grafts; bypass operation; bypass transplantation; bypass grafting	搭桥手术；心脏搭桥手术；旁路手术；旁路转流术；血管旁路转流术；血管旁路术；旁路移植术
C reactive protein; high-sensitivity C-reactive protein; C-reactive protein; hsCRP; CRP	C反应蛋白
c-Jun N-terminal kinases MAPK signaling pathway; JNK signaling pathway	c-jun N端激酶MAPK信号通路
Cabbage; cabbages	甘蓝；白菜；小白菜；大白菜；卷心菜；包菜
calcium channel blockers; calcium channel blocker; calcium channal blocker; calcium antagonist; calcium chennel blockers	钙离子拮抗剂；钙通道阻滞药；钙拮抗剂；钙通道拮抗剂；钙离子通道拮抗剂；钙通道阻滞剂
Calpain 1	钙蛋白酶1；钙激活蛋白酶1；钙依赖中性蛋白酶1
Canadian neurological scale; CNS; Central nervous system; central nervous system	加拿大神经量表；中枢神经系统；加拿大神经医学评分
Cancellation test; write off test; write off experiment; write off experiments	划消测验；划销试验；取消测验；划字测验；数字划消试验；划消试验；划销测验
Capillary malformation arteriovenous malformation; CM-AVM	毛细血管畸形动静脉畸形
Capsular warning syndrome	内囊预警综合征
Carbohydrate; Dietary carbohydrates; Carbohydrates; Carbohydrase; carbohydrate	碳水化合物；碳水化物
carbonic anhydrase IV; CA4	IV型碳酸酐酶

续 表

英文术语	中文术语
Cardiac arrest; cardiac arrest; asystole; Asystole; Cardiac arrest (disorder); Asystole (disorder)	心脏骤停；心脏停搏；心搏停止；心跳骤停；心跳停止；心搏骤停；心脏停止搏动；心跳停搏
Cardiac arrhythmia; cardiac arrhythmia; arrhythmia; Arrhythmia; Cardiac arrhythmia (disorder); Conduction disorder of the heart; Disorder of heart rhythm; Cardiac dysrhythmias; Cardiac arrhythmias; Cardiac dysrhythmia; Disorder of heart conduction; Conduction disorder of the heart (disorder)	心律失常；心律紊乱；心律不齐；心脏心律失常；心脏心律障碍；心脏节律障碍；心脏传导紊乱；心脏传导障碍
Cardiac Monitoring; cardiac care unit; cardiac monitoring; cardiac care; cardiac intensive care; heart function monitoring; heart monitor	心电监测；心脏监测；胎心监测；心脏监护；胎心监护
Caregiver support; care-taker support; caregivers support; care-taker support degree; caregivers support degree; Caregiver support degree	陪护者支持；看护者支持度；照顾者支持
Caregivers; caregiver; guardian; keeper; custodies; caretaker; guardians	看护人员；照顾者；照料者；照护者；亲属照护者；看护人；护理员；护工
Carotenoids	类胡萝卜素；类胡萝卜素类；类胡萝卜素化合物；花青素；胡萝卜素类；胡萝卜素
Carotid artery; Carotid arteries; carotid	颈动脉；颈动脉的
Carotid artery atherosclerosis; carotid atherosclerosis; Carotid atherosclerosis; Carotid artery atheroma; Carotid atherosclerosis (disorder); Carotid artery atherosclerotic plaque	颈动脉粥样硬化；颈动脉硬化；颈动脉粥样硬化斑块；颈动脉动脉粥样硬化；颈动脉硬化症；颈动脉粥样斑块；颈动脉粥样硬化斑块形成
Carotid artery dissection; carotid dissection; carotid artery dissection; Common carotid artery dissection; Carotid artery dissections; Carotid dissections; Carotid dissection	颈动脉夹层；颈总动脉夹层
Carotid artery embolism; Carotid artery thrombosis; Carotid artery thrombosis (disorder); Carotid artery embolism (disorder)	颈动脉栓塞；颈动脉血栓形成；颈动脉血栓；颈动脉血栓栓塞
Carotid artery stenosis; Asymptomatic carotid artery stenosis; Asymptomatic carotid stenosis; Carotid artery stenoses; Carotid stenosis; Carotid stenoses; Carotid artery narrowing; Carotid artery stenosis (disorder); carotid artery stenosis	颈动脉狭窄；颈动脉狭小

英文术语	中文术语
Carotid Duplex ultrasound; CDUS; neck vascular color doppler ultrasound; cervical vascular color doppler ultrasound; neck vascular ultrasound; cervical vascular ultrasound; carotid vascular color doppler ultrasound	颈部血管彩超；颈部血管彩色超声多普勒；颈动脉血管超声；颈动脉彩超
Carotid endarterectomy; CEA	颈动脉内膜剥脱术；颈动脉内膜切除术；颈内动脉内膜剥脱术；内膜剥脱术；颈动脉内膜剥除术；颈动脉内膜剥离术
Carotid Intima Media Thickness; Carotid intimal medial thickness; Carotid intimal-medial thickness; Carotid Intima-Media Thickness; CIMT	颈动脉内膜增厚
Carotid revascularization; Endovascular revascularization; Revascularization; revascularization	颈内血管重建术；血管重建；颈动脉血运重建
Carotid sinus syncope; Carotid sinus syndrome; Carotid sinus syncope (disorder); cervical syncope; carotid sinus syncope	颈动脉窦性晕厥(颈性晕厥)；颈动脉窦性晕厥；Friedmann血管舒缩综合征；颈动脉窦综合征；Charcot-Weiss-Baker综合征；Weiss—Baker综合征；颈动脉窦综合症；血管舒缩性晕厥；颈动脉窦晕厥
Carotid siphon atherosclerosis; carotid siphon arteriosclerosis; carotid siphon atherosclerotic; carotid siphon atheromatous; carotid siphon artery atherosclerosis; carotid siphon aortic atherosclerosis; carotid siphon accelerated atherosclerosis; Carotid siphon atherosclerotic plaque	颈动脉虹吸部动脉粥样硬化；颈动脉虹吸部粥样硬化斑块
Carotid sonography; carotid artery ultrasound; carotid ultrasonography; carotid artery ultrasonography; carotid sonography; carotid ultrasonic	颈动脉超声；颈动脉超声检查
Caspase 3	半胱胺酸天冬氨酸蛋白酶3；半胱氨酸天冬氨酸3；半胱氨酶3；半胱天冬酶3
Caspase independed cell death	半胱天冬酶非依赖性细胞死亡；胱天蛋白酶非依赖性细胞死亡；半胱氨酸蛋白酶非依赖性细胞死亡；胱冬肽酶非依赖性细胞死亡

续　表

英文术语	中文术语
Cathepsin B; Cat B	组织蛋白酶B；组蛋白酶B；溶酶体组织蛋白酶B；半胱氨酸组织蛋白酶B；蛋白酶B；溶酶体酶B
Catherine Bergego Scale; CBS	Catherine Bergego量表
Causative Classification System; CCS; Classification system of ischemic stroke etiology	缺血性卒中病因分类系统
Cavernous angioma; Cerebral cavernous venous malformations; Cerebral cavernous malformation; Cavernous venous malformation; cavernous haemangioma; Cavernous hemangioma; cavernoma; CCM; cavernous hemangioma; cavernous angioma; angiocavernoma; Cavernous haemangioma; Cavernous hemangioma (disorder); Cavernous haemangioma (disorder)	海绵状血管瘤；脑海绵状血管畸形；海绵窦血管瘤
Cavernous sinus thrombosis	海绵窦血栓形成；海绵窦栓塞；海绵窦血栓
CC chemokine receptor 2; Receptors, CCR2	CC趋化因子受体2
CC chemokine receptor 7; CCR7	CC趋化因子受体7
CC chemokine receptors; Receptors, CCR; CCR	CC趋化因子受体
CD40 Ligand; Tumor Necrosis Factor Ligand Superfamily Member 5; CD154 Antigens; CD40L	CD40配体
CD55 molecule; CD55	CD55分子
Cell death; Cell damage	细胞死亡；细胞坏死；细胞凋亡；细胞损伤
Cellular mediator; inflammatory cellular; inflammation cell; inflammatory cell infiltration; immune cells; inflammation cells; Inflammatory cells; inflammatory cell	炎症细胞
central nervous system vasculitis; primary angiitis; Cerebral vasculitis; Cerebral angitis; CNS vasculitis; Cerebral vasculitis (disorder)	中枢神经系统血管炎；脑血管炎；脑脉管炎；脑血管炎症
central post-stroke pain; Central Pain After Stroke; central pain after stroke	卒中后中枢痛；脑卒中后中枢痛
Central scotoma; central scotoma; Scotoma of central area; Central scotoma (finding)	中心暗点；中央暗点

英文术语	中文术语
Centrocaecal scotoma; Paracentral scotoma; Paracentral scotoma (finding); Centrocecal scotoma; Cecocentral scotoma; Centrocecal scotoma (finding)	近中心性暗点；中心旁暗点；旁中心暗点；中心盲点暗点；中心盲点性暗点
Cerebellar ataxia associated with quadrupedal gait	小脑性共济失调与四足步态相关
Cerebellar infarction syndrome; syndromes of cerebellar infarction; syndrome of cerebellar infarction; Cerebellar infarction syndromes; Cerebellar infarction symptoms; Cerebellar infarction symptom	小脑梗死综合征
Cerebellum; cerebellum	小脑
Cerebral arteritis; Cerebral arteritis (disorder)	脑动脉炎；大脑动脉炎
Cerebral arteritis in Giant cell arteritis; Giant cell arteritis; Megacellular arteritis middle cerebral arteritis	巨细胞动脉炎；巨细胞动脉炎中脑动脉炎
Cerebral artery; cerebral arteries; cerebral artery	脑动脉
Cerebral artery embolism; cerebral embolism; intracranial arterial embolism	脑动脉栓塞；脑血管栓塞；脑栓塞；颅内动脉栓塞
Cerebral cavernous malformation-1; Cerebral cavernous malformation 1; CCM-1; CCM1	1型脑海绵状血管畸形
Cerebral cavernous malformation-2; Cerebral cavernous malformation 2; CCM-2; CCM2	2型脑海绵状血管畸形
Cerebral cavernous malformation-3; Cerebral cavernous malformation 3; CCM-3; CCM3	3型脑海绵状血管畸形
Cerebral edema; Brain edema; Perihematomal edema; Brain Swelling	脑水肿；弥漫性脑肿胀；脑肿胀；脑组织水肿
Cerebral hemisphere; cerebral hemisphere; Hemicephaly; Hemicephaly (disorder)	大脑半球
Cerebral hernia	脑疝
Cerebral malformation syndromes; Brain malformation syndrome	脑畸形综合征
Cerebral venous sinus thrombosis; CVST; Thrombosis of intracranial venous sinus; Central sinus thrombosis; Dural sinus thrombosis; Cerebral venous sinus thrombosis (disorder)	颅内静脉窦血栓形成；硬膜窦血栓

续　表

英文术语	中文术语
Cerebral venous thrombosis; Thrombosis of cerebral veins (disorder); Intracranial venous thrombosis; Thrombosis of cerebral vein; Cerebral vein thrombosis; CVT; Thrombosis of cerebral veins; cerebral vein thrombosis; intracranial venous thrombosis; cerebral venous sinus thrombosis; Intracranial venous thrombosis (disorder)	颅内静脉系统血栓形成；脑静脉血栓；脑静脉血栓栓塞；脑静脉栓塞；脑静脉血栓形成；颅内静脉血栓形成；颅内静脉血栓栓塞；颅内静脉血栓；颅内静脉栓塞
cerebrovascular spasm; Intracranial Vasospasm; cerebral angiospasm ; cerebral vascular spasm ; brain vascular spasm; cerebral vessels spasm; cerebral vessel spasm; cerebral arterial vasospasm; Cerebral vasospasm	脑血管痉挛；颅内血管痉挛；血管收缩
Cerovive; disufenton sodium; NXY-059	地舒芬通钠
Cervical artery dissection; cervical artery interlayer; Arterial dissection	颈部动脉夹层；动脉夹层
CETP inhibitors; cholesteryl ester transfer protein inhibitors; cetp inhibitors; cholesterol ester transfer protein inhibitor	胆固醇酯转移蛋白抑制剂；胆固醇转运蛋白抑制；CETP抑制剂
Charlson Comorbidity Index; CCI	察尔森合并症指数
Chedoke Arm and Hand Activity Inventory; CAHAI	切多克手臂和手部活动清单；Chedoke手臂和手部活动清单
Chedoke McMaster Stroke Assessment	切多克•麦克马斯特中风评估；Chedoke McMaster中风评估
chemical-induced vasculitis; chemical injuries vasculitis; chemical-induced vessel vasculitis; chemical vessel vasculitis; chemical injuries vessel vasculitis; chemical-induced angiitis; chemical angiitis; chemical injuries angiitis; Chemical vasculitis	化学物质诱导的血管炎；化学性血管炎
chemokine (C-C motif) ligand 2 signaling pathway; Ccl2 signaling pathway	趋化因子（C-C基序）配体2信号通路
Cheyne-Stokes respiration; Cheyne Stokes breathing; cheyne-stokes respiration	潮式呼吸；斯托克斯呼吸；Cheyne-Stokes呼吸
Chin myoclonus	下颌肌阵挛
Chinese Ischemic Stroke Subclassification; china ischemic stroke subtype ; china ischemic stroke subclassification ; chinese ischemic stroke subtype; chinese ischemic strock subclassification ; chinese ischemic stroke subclassification ; CISS	中国缺血性卒中亚型
Chocolate; chocolates	巧克力

英文术语	中文术语
Cholesterol metabolism; cholesterol homeostasis; cholesterol catabolism; lipid metabolism; cholesterin; cholesterol synthesis	胆固醇代谢
Cholesteryl ester; cholesterol ester	胆固醇酯；总胆固醇酯；胆甾醇酯
Cholesteryl ester transfer protein; CETP	胆固醇酯转移蛋白；胆固醇脂转运蛋白；胆固醇转运脂蛋白；胆固醇酯转运蛋白
chondroitin sulfate proteoglycan 2; CSPG2; VCAN	硫酸软骨素蛋白聚糖2
Chorea; Ballism; chorea; Dance-like; ballism; Choreaform movement; Choreiform movement; Choreic movement; Chorea (finding); Ballism (disorder)	舞蹈病；舞蹈样运动；投掷症；舞蹈症；舞蹈病样运动；舞蹈病运动；舞蹈病性运动；舞蹈症样运动
Choreiform dyskinesias	舞蹈样运动障碍；舞蹈病样的运动障碍
Choreoathetoid movements	舞蹈样手足徐动症；舞蹈手足徐动症；手足徐动症
Choreoathetosis; choreoathetosis; CHOREOATHETOSIS; Choreoathetosis (disorder)	舞蹈手足徐动症；舞蹈样手足徐动；舞蹈徐动症
Chronic hypertension; chronic high blood pressure	慢性高血压；缓进型高血压病；慢性静脉窦高压；慢性高血压病
chronic kidney disease; Chronic Renal Disease; Chronic renal failure; Chronic renal failure syndrome; CRF - Chronic renal failure; Chronic renal failure syndrome (disorder); Chronic renal disease; Chronic kidney disease (disorder); chronic kidney insufficiency; chronic kidney insufficiencies; Chronic kidney disease; CKD	慢性肾病；慢性肾脏病；慢性肾疾病；慢性肾功能衰竭；慢性肾衰竭综合征；慢性肾衰竭；慢性肾脏功能衰竭；慢性肾衰综合征；慢性肾脏疾病
Churg-strauss syndrome; Allergic angitis and granulomatosis	变应性肉芽肿性血管炎；嗜酸性肉芽肿性多血管炎；变应性肉芽肿综合征；变应性血管炎和肉芽肿病
Cilostazol; cilostazol tablets	西洛他唑；西洛他唑片
Circulating adhesion molecules; Circulating adhesion molecule; Adhesion molecules; Adhesion molecule	循环粘附分子
Citicoline; Cytidine Diphosphate Choline; citicoline	胞二磷胆碱；胞磷胆械碱
Citrus fruit; Citrus	柑橘果实；柑橘；柑桔；柑桔类水果；柑桔果实；柑橘类鲜果

续　表

英文术语	中文术语
Classification of atherosclerotic cerebrovascular diseases; Model of Atherosclerotic Cerebrovascular Disease; Classification of atherosclerotic cerebrovascular disease	动脉粥样硬化性脑血管疾病分型
Claude syndrome; Claude's syndrome; Claude's syndrome (disorder)	克劳德综合征；Claude综合征；克劳德综合征(一侧动眼神经麻痹、对侧不能协同合并讷吃)；克洛德综合征
Clinical Manifestation; Clinical Situation; clinical presentation; clinical features; clinical feature	临床表现；临床特点；临床特征；临床症状
Clinical Memory Test; clinical memory scales; clinical memory scale	临床记忆量表；临床记忆测验
Clomethiazole	氯美噻唑
Clopidogrel; Plavix; clopidogrel sulfate; chlorine clopidogrel; hydrochloride; clopidogrel hydrogen	氯吡格雷；硫酸氢氯吡格雷；氯吡咯雷；氢氯吡格雷；氯吡格雷；硫酸氢吡格雷
Cluster headache; cluster headache; Histamine headache; Histamine cephalgia; Cluster headache syndrome; Vasomotor headache; Cluster headache syndrome (disorder)	丛集性头痛；集束性头痛；丛集性头痛综合征；组胺性头痛；血管舒缩性头痛；霍顿氏头痛；从集性头痛；组织胺性头痛；组胺头痛
Coagulation disorder; Inherited hematological abnormalities; Inherited hematological abnormality; Blood coagulation disorder; Coagulopathy; Disorder of hemostasis; Disorder of haemostasis	凝血障碍；血液凝固障碍；止血障碍；血凝固障碍；血凝固病症；凝血功能异常
coagulation factor inhibitors; Antithrombotic proteins	抗凝蛋白异常；抗凝蛋白
coagulation factor V; Factor V; F5	凝血因子V
coagulation factor ⅩⅢ a; F13A1	凝血因子ⅩⅢ a
Coca alkaloid; theobromine	可可碱；古柯碱；生物碱
Cocaine hydrochloride; cocaine; Cocaine	可卡因；古柯碱
Cocoa	可可；可可粉
Coexist risk factor medications; Drugs for coexisting risk factors	共存危险因素药物；共存危险因素用药；并存危险因素用药；并存风险因素用药
Coffee intake; consumption of coffee	咖啡摄入量；咖啡摄入

英文术语	中文术语
Cognitive ability to participate in rehabilitation treatment; Cognitive abilities to participate in rehabilitation therapy; cognitive abilities to attendance rehabilitation therapy	参加康复治疗的认知能力；参与康复治疗的认知
Cognitive and behavioral disturbance	认知和行为障碍
Cognitive disturbance; Cognitive deficit; Cognitive dysfunction	认知功能障碍
Cognitive function retraining; Cognitive functions retraining; cognition function retraining; cognitive impairment retraining; cognitive function impairment retraining; cognitive ability retraining; cognitive retraining; Cognitive function reeducation; Cognitive functions reeducation; cognitive ability reeducation; cognitive reeducation; cognition function reeducation; cognitive impairment reeducation; cognitive function impairment reeducation	认知功能再训练；认知功能再培训
Cold massage induced swallowing test	冷按摩引发吞咽测试；冷按摩诱导吞咽试验
Colestipol	考来替泊；降脂宁；降脂2号树脂
Colestyramine; Cholestyramine resin	考来烯胺；消胆胺
Collagen type Ⅳ A1 associated vasculopathy; Type Ⅳ collagen A1 - related vascular lesions	Ⅳ A1型胶原相关性血管病；Ⅳ型胶原A1相关血管病变
collagen type Ⅳ alpha 1; COL4A1	Ⅳ型胶原 α1
collagen type Ⅳ alpha 2; COL4A2	Ⅳ型胶原 α2
Collier's sign; Collier sign	Collier's 征；Collier 标志
color doppler ultrasound; color doppler ultrasonography	彩色多普勒超声；彩色多普勒超声探查
Coma; coma; Comatose; Exanimation; Coma (disorder)	昏迷；昏迷状态
Combined duplex and Transcranial Doppler; Combined duplex and TCD	联合双频和经颅多普勒；双频和经颅多普勒联合检查
Combined intravenous-intraarterial thrombolysis; Combined IV/IA Thrombolysis	联合静脉-动脉内溶栓；静脉-动脉内联合溶栓
Common carotid artery; Common carotid arteries; CCAs; CCA; arteria carotis communis; common carotid artery	颈总动脉
communication disorders; communication obstacle; communication barrier; communication barriers; communication impairments; communication disorder; communicative barriers; impaired communication; Communication Impairment	沟通障碍；交流障碍

续　表

英文术语	中文术语
communication function; communicative function	沟通功能；交际功能；交流功能
communicative activities in daily living; CADL	日常生活交往活动检查；日常生活中的交际活动
Community rehabilitation institutions; Community rehabilitation mechanism; Community rehabilitation organization; Community rehabilitation institution; community recovery mechanism; community recovery organization; community recovery institution	社区康复机构
Community support; community supporting; community supports; community adaptation; community's support	社区支持；社区支持度；社区帮扶；社区保障；社区支持感
Comorbidity; Comorbidities of stroke; Comorbidity of stroke; Stroke comorbidities; Stroke comorbidity; Co-morbidities; Comorbidities; Co-morbidity	合并症；中风并发症；共病
Comorbidity severity index; Comorbidity-severity index	共病严重程度指数
Complement C3	补体C3；补体C3基因；补体成分C3
Complete blood count; CBC; complete blood cell count	全血细胞计数；全部血细胞数；血细胞计数；全部血细胞计数
Complex hyperkinesias	复杂运动过度；复合运动亢进
Complication; complication; complications; Complication of stroke; Stroke complications; Stroke complication; Complications; Complication (disorder)	并发症；卒中并发症
Composite Spasticity Index; CSI	综合痉挛指数
Comprehensive stroke center; CSCU; CSC; Comprehensive Stroke Care Unit	综合卒中中心；高级卒中中心
Computerized Tomography; computed tomography; CT; computerized tomography; CT; Computerized tomography scan; Computed tomography; Brain CT scan; CT scans; Brain CT; CT scan	电子计算机断层扫描；计算机体层摄影；计算机断层扫描；ct扫描；ct表现；ct检查；ct螺旋
Confusion; Clouding of consciousness; clouding of consciousness; confusion; Clouded consciousness; CONFUSION; Clouded consciousness (finding)	意识模糊；意识混浊
Congenital bilateral ptosis; Congenital Bilateral eyelid ptosis; Congenital double sides ptosis; Congenital two-sided ptosis	先天性双侧上睑下垂；先天性两侧上睑下垂

续　表

英文术语	中文术语
Congenital horizontal nystagmus; Congenital horizontal tremor; Congenital horizontal eyeball tremor	先天性水平眼震；先天性水平性眼球震颤
Congenital Horner syndrome; congenital Bernard-Horner syndrome; congenital Claude-Bernard-Horner syndrome ; congenital horner syndrome; congenital horner's syndrome	先天性霍纳综合征
Congenital miosis; Congenital miosis (disorder)	先天性瞳孔缩小
Congenital nystagmus; congenital nystagmus; Congenital nystagmus (disorder)	先天性眼球震颤；先天性眼震；先天性遗传性眼球震颤；先天眼震
Congenital ptosis; congenital ptosis; congenital blepharoptosis; Congenital ptosis (disorder); Congenital dysgenetic ptosis; Congenital dysgenetic ptosis (disorder)	先天性上睑下垂；先天性上眼睑下垂；先天遗传性上睑下垂；遗传性上睑下垂
Congruous heteronymous hemianopia; Consistent lateral blindness; Consistent heteronymous	一致性对侧偏盲；一致性交叉性偏盲
Congruous homonymous hemianopia; Consistent homolateral blinding; Consistent equilateral hemianopia	一致性同侧偏盲；一致性同向偏盲；一致性同向性偏盲
Conjugate eye deviation; Conjugated visual deviation; Conjugated visual deviation (finding)	眼球同向偏视；同向偏视
Conjugate gaze paresis; Conjugate gaze palsies	共轭凝视轻瘫；共轭注视轻瘫
Connective tissue disorder; Disorder of connective tissue; Connective tissue disease; Disease of connective tissues; Disease of connective tissues (disorder); Disorder of connective tissue (disorder)	结缔组织疾病；结缔组织病；结缔组织病变
Consciousness; consciousness; conscious	意识清晰；有意识
consciousness; awareness; sense; conscious	意识；意识状态
Constant velocity shooting test	等速拍击试验；恒速射击试验
Constipation; CONSTIPATION; constipation; CN - Constipation; Constipated; Constipation (disorder); Constipation (finding)	便秘；大便秘结；便秘待查；便秘(粪便嵌塞除外)
Constraint indused therapy; Constraint induction therapy	约束诱导运动疗法；约束介入治疗；约束诱导疗法
constraint-induced language therapy; CILT	强制性诱导失语症治疗；强制性诱导语言治疗

续　表

英文术语	中文术语
constraint-induced movement therapy; Compulsory exercise therapy; Compulsory exercise treatment; constrained motion treatment; Compulsory exercise therapeutics; constrained motion therapeutics; constrained motion therapy	强制性诱导运动治疗；强制性运动疗法
Constricted visual fields; stenosis visual field; narrowing visual field; narrow visual field; contraction visual field; stenosis vision; narrowing vision; narrow vision; contraction vision	视野狭窄；狭窄视野
constructional apraxia; Constructive aphasia; Structural apraxia	结构性失用；构念性失用；构念性运用不能；结构性失用症
consumers' education; comsumer education; succoring consumers; education of consumers	用户教育；消费者教育；顾客教育；患者教育
Continuous shoulder joint activity training; Continuous shoulder range of motion training; Continuous shoulder mobility training; Continuous shoulder joint mobility training; Continuous range of motion of shoulder joint training; lasting shoulder range of motion training; lasting shoulder mobility training; lasting shoulder joint mobility training; lasting range of motion of shoulder joint training	连续肩关节活动训练；持续肩关节活动度训练
Contralateral facial paralysis; Lateral paralysis; Contralateral facial palsy ; Contralateral paralysis facialis; Contralateral hemiparesis sparing the face	对侧面瘫
Contralateral fourth cranial nerve palsy	对侧第四颅神经麻痹
Contralateral hemihypesthesia	对侧偏身感觉障碍；对侧偏身感觉减退；对侧偏身感觉迟钝
Contralateral hemihypesthesia with mild hemiparesis; Contralateral hemisensory loss with mild hemiparesis	对侧偏身感觉障碍伴轻偏瘫；对侧半感觉丧失伴轻度偏瘫
Contralateral hemiplegia; Contralateral hemiparesis; Contralateral hemiparesis with cognitive disturbance	对侧偏瘫；对侧轻偏瘫；对侧偏侧不全麻痹
Contralateral hyperkinetic movements; Jerky dystonic unsteady hand syndrom	对侧运动过度；对侧亢进运动；对侧运动亢进
Contralateral lemniscal sensory loss; Paravertebral sensory loss	对侧丘系感觉障碍；对侧椎板感觉丧失；对侧丘系感觉丧失；对侧椎板感觉障碍
Contralateral limb ataxia; Contralateral appendicular ataxia	对侧肢体共济失调；对侧肢体运动失调

英文术语	中文术语
Contralateral motor disorders; Contralateral movement disorders; Contralateral motor dysfunction; Contralateral motility disorders; Contralateral motor disorder; Contralateral motor disturbance; Contralateral disturbance of motion; Contralateral motor deficit	对侧肢体运动障碍；对侧运动功能障碍；对侧运动障碍
Contralateral thermoalgesic deficit; Impaired thermal sensitivity; Contralateral thermalgesia	对侧痛温觉减退；热敏度受损；对侧热痛觉缺陷；对侧热痛觉障碍
Contralateral visual field neglect; Neglect of opposite view	对侧忽视；对侧视野忽略
contrast bath; alternating hot and cold bath	冷热交替浴
Contrast Enhanced MRA; Contrast-enhanced Magnetic Resonance Imaging; CE MRA	对比增强MRA
Control ability of defecation; Defecation control ability	排便控制能力；大小便控制能力
Controlateral sensory deficit; Control-side sensory disturbance; Control-side sensory deficit; Controlateral sensory disturbance	对侧感觉障碍；控制性感觉缺陷；控制性感觉障碍
Conventional angiography; conventional catheter-based angiography	常规血管造影；常规冠状动脉造影；普通血管造影
Conventional magnetic resonance imaging; Conventional MRI	常规磁共振成像
cook; prepare a meal	做饭；煮饭；烹调；烹饪
Corneal hypesthesia; Corneal sensory disturbance; Corneal sensation disorders; Corneal sensation disorder; Corneal sensation disturbance	角膜感觉减退；角膜感觉迟钝；角膜知觉减退
Cortex; cortex	皮层；皮质；脑皮质
Cortical blindness syndrome; Anton's syndrome; Blindsight	皮质盲综合征
Cortical deafness	皮层耳聋；大脑皮质性聋；皮质聋；皮质性聋
cortical myoclonus	皮质性肌阵挛
Cortical vein thrombosis; Superficial vein thrombosis; Superficial vein thrombosis (disorder)	皮层静脉血栓形成；浅静脉血栓形成；浅表性静脉血栓形成
CR1; CD35	补体受体1
Crack cocaine; Strong cocaine	强效可卡因；快克可卡因
Craniofacial dystonia	头面部肌张力障碍
Creamed products	奶油产品；奶油制品

续　表

英文术语	中文术语
Crossed hemiataxia; Cross-biased ataxia; Crossed hemiataxy	交叉性偏身共济失调；交叉性偏身运动失调；交叉性半共济失调
Crossed hemihypesthesia; Cross-offset sensation decreased	交叉偏身感觉减退；交叉偏身感觉迟钝；交叉偏身感觉障碍
Cruciferous vegetables; Cruciferous vegetable	十字花科蔬菜；十字花蔬菜
cryotherapy; cold therapy	冷疗法；冷疗
CT angiography; Computerized tomography angiography; Computed tomography angiography; CTA	CT血管成像；血管造影CT；血管成像；放射CT血管造影；CT血管造影
Cumulative illness rating scale; Cumulative Disease Rating Scale	累积疾病评定量表
Cytochrome c; CytC; CYC	细胞色素C；细胞色素C类
Cytokine; cytokine; Cytokines	细胞因子；细胞因子素
Cytokines biomarkers; proinflamamtory and anti-inflammatory cytokines biomarkers; anti-inflammatory cytokines; proinflamamtory cytokines; Cytokine biomarkers; Cytokines biomarker	细胞因子生物标志物
cytoskeleton-associated protein 4; CKAP4	细胞骨架蛋白4
Cytotoxic edema; Oncotic cell swelling; Cellular edema; Oncosis	细胞毒性水肿；细胞性水肿；肿瘤病；肿瘤细胞肿胀
D-Dimer; D dimer	D-二聚体
Dabigatran	达比加群酯
Death; Stroke-related mortality; Hemorrhagic stroke death; Ischemic stroke death; Stroke death; Mortality	死亡；猝死
decompressive craniectomy; Decompressive Surgery; decompressive craniotomy	去骨瓣减压术；大骨瓣手术；减压手术
decompressor; decompression device; pressure reducing device; relief device; pressure relief fitting	减压装置；减压器；降压装置
Decubitus	褥疮

英文术语	中文术语
Deep venous thrombosis; Deep vein thrombosis; Deep-vein thrombosis; DVT; deep venous thrombosis; DVT - Deep vein thrombosis; Deep venous thrombosis (disorder); Deep venous thrombosis of lower extremity; Deep vein thrombosis of lower limb; Deep venous thrombosis of lower limb; DVT - Deep vein thrombosis of lower limb; Deep venous thrombosis of leg; Deep venous thrombosis of lower extremity (disorder)	深静脉血栓形成；深部静脉血栓形成；深静脉血栓；下肢深静脉血栓形成；下肢深静脉栓塞；下肢深静脉血栓
Defibrogenating Enzymes; degrading enzyme; degradation enzyme; degrading enzymes; degradation enzymes; degraded enzyme; degradative enzyme	降解酶；去纤化酶
Deficiency of protein C; Protein C deficiency disease; Protein C deficiency disease (disorder); Protein C deficiency	蛋白C缺乏症；C蛋白缺乏病；蛋白质C缺乏；蛋白C缺乏症
Deficiency of protein S; S protein deficiency disease; protein S deficiency	蛋白质S缺乏；S蛋白缺乏病
Deficiency of antithrombin Ⅲ; Antithrombin Ⅲ Deficiency; Antithrombin Ⅲ deficiency; glycoprotein antithrombin; Antithrombin deficiency; Antithombin Ⅲ deficiency; Antithrombin 3 deficiency; AT deficiency - Antithrombin deficiency; Antithrombin Ⅲ deficiency (disorder)	抗凝血酶Ⅲ缺乏；抗凝血酶Ⅲ缺乏；抗凝血酶原Ⅲ缺乏症；抗凝血酶Ⅲ缺乏
Delirium; delirium; Acute brain syndrome; Delirium (disorder)	谵妄；急性脑病；谵妄状态；妄想综合征
Dementia; cognitive disorder; Cognitive Disorder; dementia; Cognitive impairment; Cognitive disorder; Dementia (disorder); Cognitive disorder (disorder); Impaired cognition; Cognitive decline; Impaired cognition (finding)	认知障碍；痴呆；认知损害；认知减退；认知能力下降 ；认知能力衰退
Depression; Depressive Disorders; Depressive Disorder; depression; Depressive disorder; Depressed; Depressive illness; Depressive episode; Depressive disorder (disorder)	抑郁症；抑郁；精神忧郁症；抑郁病；忧郁症
Desmoteplase	德斯莫替普酶
Deuteranomoly; deuteranomalia	绿色弱视；绿色弱
Deuteranopia; deuteranopia; deuteranopsia	绿色盲；第二型色盲；第二原色盲
Dexamethasone; dexamethasone	地塞米松；氟甲强的松龙
Dextrorphan	右啡烷；右羟吗喃；去甲基右美沙芬；去甲氢溴酸右美沙芬

续　表

英文术语	中文术语
Diabetes mellitus; Diabetes; DM; Dermatomyositis; dermatomyositis; Diabetes mellitus (disorder); diabetes mellitus; diabetes; Diabetes Mellitus; DM - Dermatomyositis; Dermatomyositis (disorder)	糖尿病；皮肌炎
Diagnosis; Diagnostic; Diagnosed; Dx; diagnosis	诊断
Diagnosis cost group; Diagnosis cost groups; DCGs; DCG	诊断费用组
Diagnostic evaluation; Diagnostic evaluations	诊断性评估；诊断性评价；诊断评估；诊断性测评
Diagnostic tests; Diagnostic test	诊断测试；诊断试验
Dichromacy; Doublechromatic blindness; Doublechromatic blind; two-colour blindness; two-color blindness	双色盲；两色盲
Dietary Approaches to Stop Hypertension diet; DASH-style diets; DASH diet	控制高血压饮食的饮食方法；低盐低脂饮食
Dietary cholesterol; cholesterol	膳食胆固醇；胆固醇
Dietary factor; Nutritional factors; Nutritional factor; Dietary factors; Diet factors	饮食因素；膳食因素；食物要素；食物因素
Dietary habit; Dietary habits; Food Habit	饮食习惯；膳食习惯；日常饮食；饮食行为
Dietary intake; diet; dietary; meal; dietary intake; nutrition	饮食摄入；膳食；摄入食物；饮食；进食量；膳食调查；饮食摄入量
Dietary pattern; dietary patterns; pattern of diet; dietary model; meals pattern	膳食模式；饮食模式；膳食构成；日粮模式；膳食类型
Differential diagnosis; DDx	鉴别诊断
Diffusion weighted magnetic resonance imaging; Diffusion weighted imaging; Diffusion weighted MRI; DWI	磁共振弥散加权成像
Digital Imaging Inspection; digital radiographic Inspection; digital image Inspection; digital photography Inspection; digital radiography Inspection	数字成像检查；数字影像检测；数字造影检测；数字化影像检测
Diplopia; diplopia; DIPLOPIA; Double vision; Diplopia (disorder)	复视；复视觉
Dipyridamole with aspirin; Dipyridamole+aspirin; Aggrenox	阿司匹林双嘧达莫片
Directional force problem; directive force problem; directive force problems; directive force issues; directive force issue	定向力障碍

英文术语	中文术语
Disability; Disabilities; disability; Disability (finding)	致残；残疾；失能；病废；残疾人；劳动能力丧失；功能障碍
Disability Assessment Scale; DAS	残疾评估量表
disruption of Brain blood barrier; Brain blood barrier disruption; Loss of blood brain barrier integrity; breakdown of Brain blood barrier; Blood brain barrier disruption; Brain blood barrier breakdown; Loss of blood brain barrier; Loss of BBB integrity; Blood brain barriers; Blood-brain barriers; Brain blood barriers; Blood brain barrier; Blood-brain barrier; BBB disruption; Loss of BBB	血脑屏障破坏；脑血屏障破坏；血脑屏障；血脑屏障完整性丧失
Dissociated nystagmus; Divergence nystagmus; dissociated nystagmus; Dissociated nystagmus (disorder)	分离性眼震；散开性眼震；分离性眼球震颤
Distal limb weakness ; Weakness of distal lower limb; Contralateral weakness of lower extremity	下肢远端无力；下肢远端虚弱
DNA fragmentation; DNA cleavage; DNA fragment; DNA strand breaks; DNA damage; DNA strand break; DNA breakages; DNA breaks	DNA断裂；DNA电泳；DNA琼脂糖；DNA降解；DNA断片；DNA大片段化；DNA断片化；DNA片段
Double lip training; Double lip exercise; Double lip train	双唇训练
Downbeat nystagmus; Down beat nystagmus; Downbeat central vestibular nystagmus; Downbeat central nystagmus; Downbeat nystagmus (disorder); Downbeat central vestibular nystagmus (disorder)	下跳性眼球震颤；下击型眼球震颤；下视性眼球震颤
Drawing Experiment; paint experiments; drawing test; graph drawing test; graph drawing experiment; graph drawing experiments; paint experiment	绘图测试；画图试验；手绘实验；绘图实验
dressing; to dress oneself; dress; overcoat	穿衣；穿衣服
Drink intake; Beverage intake; beverages intake; drinks intake; juices intake; beverage processing intake; soft drinks	饮料摄入
Drug-induced vasculitis; Drug induced vasculitis; Drug induced vessel vasculitis; Drug-induced angiitis	药物诱导的血管炎；药源性血管炎
dual antiplatelet therapy with clopidogrel-aspirin; Clopidogrel-aspirin; Dual clopidogrel aspirin; Clopidogrel aspirin; DAPT	氯吡格雷-阿司匹林双联抗血小板治疗
dual specificity phosphatase 5; DUSP5	双特异性磷酸酶5

续　表

英文术语	中文术语
Durable Medical Devices; durable medical equipment	耐用医疗设备；耐用医疗器械
Dural venous sinus thrombosis; dural sinus thrombosis	硬脑膜静脉窦血栓形成；硬脑膜静脉窦血管栓塞
Dynamic pressure pad; active pressure pad; active pressure cushion; Dynamic pressure cushion; Dynamic pressure pads	动压垫；动态压力垫
dynorphin; Increase of dynorphin	强啡呔；强啡肽；达脑啡肽；强腓肽
Dysarthria clumsy hand syndrome; dysarthria-clumsy hand syndrome; Dysarthria-clumsy hand syndrome; Dysarthria-clumsy hand syndrome (disorder)	构音困难手笨拙综合征
Dyschromatopsia; Impairment of colour vision; dyschromatopsia; Abnormality of color vision	色觉障碍
Dysdiadochokinesis; dysdiadochokinesia; Dysdiadochokinesia; Dysdiadokokinesia; Dysdiadokokinesis; Dysdiadochokinesis (finding)	轮替运动障碍；轮替运动困难；轮替动作困难
Dysesthesia; Dysaesthesia; Dysesthesia (abnormal sensation); Dysaesthesia (abnormal sensation); Dysesthesia (finding)	感觉迟钝；触物感痛；感觉不良
Dysfibrinogenemia; hereditary dysfibrinogenemia; dysfibrinogenemia; Hereditary dysfibrinogenaemia; Congenital dysfibrinogenaemia; Hereditary dysfibrinogenemia (disorder); Congenital dysfibrinogenemia (disorder); Hereditary dysfibrinogenemia; Congenital dysfibrinogenemia; Dysfibrinogenaemia; Dysfibrinogenemia (disorder)	异常纤维蛋白原血症；遗传性异常纤维蛋白原血症；先天性异常纤维蛋白原血症；异常纤维蛋白原血症(先天性)
Dyslipidemia; Dyslipoproteinemias; Dyslipoproteinemia; Dyslipidemias; dyslipidemia; Dyslipidaemia; Dyslipidemia (disorder)	脂蛋白代谢紊乱；血脂异常；血脂紊乱；异常血脂症；脂代谢紊乱；脂代谢异常
dysmasesia; Chewing difficulties; bradymasesis; dysmasesis	吞咽困难；咀嚼障碍
Dysmetria; dysmetria; Dysmetria (finding)	辨距不良；辨距困难
Dysmnesia; Impaired memory; Memory impairment; Disturbance of memory; Memory deficit; Memory dysfunction; Memory impairment (finding)	记忆障碍；记忆损害
Dysphagia; dysphagia; Difficulty in swallowing; Dysphagia (disorder); Swallowing difficult; Impaired swallowing	吞咽障碍；吞咽困难；咽食困难

英文术语	中文术语
Dysphonia; Difficulty speaking; Disorder of speech; Disorder of voice; Difficulty speaking (disorder); Inability to produce voice sounds; dysphonia	发声困难；发音困难；发声障碍
dysplasminogenemia; Plasminogen abnormality; Plasminogen aberrant; Plasminogen disorder	纤溶酶原异常症
Dyspraxia; dyspraxia; Dyspraxia (finding); Alien Hand Syndrome	失用
Dyssynergia; dyssynergia	协同失调；协同动作障碍
Dystonia; Dystonic disorders; dysmyotonia; dystonia; myodystonia; Dystonic Disorders; Dystonia disorder; Dystonia (disorder)	肌张力障碍综合征；肌张力障碍；肌张力障碍综合症；肌张力异常；肌张力异常综合征
E-Selectin; Endothelial Leukocyte Adhesion Molecule -1; Endothelial Leukocyte Adhesion Molecule 1; E Selectin; ELAM-1	E选择素；内皮白细胞黏附分子1
Eales disease; Eales's disease; Eales' disease (disorder); Eales' disease	Eales病；视网膜静脉周围炎(Eales病)；视网膜血管周炎；视网膜血管周围炎；视网膜静脉周围炎；伊耳斯氏病；伊耳斯病；伊耳斯病<Eale's>
Eating; intake; intake, food; food intake; alimentation; diet ; meals	进食；吃
Edaravon	依达拉奉
Edoxaban	艾多沙班；依杜沙班；甲苯磺酸依度沙班水合物
Education; Educational Intervention; Education Intervention	教育；教学；培养
Ehlers Danlos syndrome type IV; Ehlers-Danlos syndrome; Cutis hyperelastica; Cutis elastica; Cutis hyperelastica dermatorrhexis; Danlos disease; Meekeren-Ehlers-Danlos syndrome; Ehlers-Danlos syndrome (disorder)	埃莱尔-当洛综合征；埃勒斯-当洛斯综合征；弹力过度性皮肤；埃勒斯-当洛综合征；Ehlers-Danlos综合征；皮肤弹性过度综合征；埃莱尔-当洛综合症；全身弹力纤维发育异常症；皮肤弹力过度综合征；Meekein-Ehlers-Danlos综合征；Danlos病；EhlersDanlos综合征；埃勒斯当洛综合征；埃勒斯当洛斯综合征；Meekeren-Ehlers-Danlos综合征；Danlos综合征
electroencepha-lographic biofeedback therapy; eeg biofeedback therapy; electroencephalographic biofeedback therapy; electroencephalogram biofeedback	脑电生物反馈疗法

续　表

英文术语	中文术语
Electroencephalography; Electroencephalogram; EEGs; EEG	脑电图；脑电描记术；脑电图描记术；脑动电流描记法；脑电图描计法
Electrolyte intake; Mineral; Minerals intake; Minerals; mineral	矿物质；无机盐
electromyogram; electromyography; quantitative electromyography; emg electromyogram; diaphragmatic electromyogram; electromyograph	肌电图；肌电描记图；肌电图检测；神经-肌电图
Electromyographic Biofeedback; myoelectric biofeedback; electromyographic biofeedback; electromyogram biofeedback; electroencephalography biofeedback; electronic biofeedback; electromyographic biofeedback treatment; emg biofeedback	肌电生物反馈；表面肌电生物反馈；电子生物反馈；肌电反馈；肌电生物反馈治疗
electromyographic biofeedback therapy; EMGBFT	肌电生物反馈疗法
Electrophysiological biomarkers of stroke	脑卒中的电生理生物标志物
Elevated hematocrit; red cell backlog Elevated; red blood cells deposited Elevated; red blood cell hematocrit Elevated	红细胞压积升高；红细胞比容升高
Elevated level of plasminogen activator inhibitor; Plasminogen activators deficiency; Plasminogen activator deficiency; PAI_1	纤溶酶原激活物抑制剂水平升高；纤溶酶原激活物缺乏
Elevated levels of factor Ⅷ; Factor Ⅷ	凝血因子Ⅷ水平升高；凝血因子Ⅷ
Elevated levels of homocysteine; Hyperhomocysteinaemia; Hyperhomocysteinemia; hyperhomocysteinemia; Hyperhomocysteinemia (disorder)	高同型半胱氨酸血症；高同种半胱胺酸血症
Elevated von willebrand factor	血管性血友病因子升高；血管外肺水指数升高；冯维尔布兰德因子升高；von Willebran因子升高；血管性血友病银子升高；血管性假学友病因子升高；血管假性性血友病因子升高
Elevation of intracellular Ca 2 pluse level; Elevation of intracellular Ca 2+ level; Increased intracellular calcium level	细胞内钙离子浓度升高；细胞内钙水平升高
Eliprodil	依利罗地
emergency department; emergency room; Emergency service; emergency departments; emergency ward; hospital emergency room; emergency	急诊科；急诊室；急诊

续　表

英文术语	中文术语
Emotional disturbance; affective symptoms; emotional obstacles; mood disorders; affective disorder; mood disorder; affective barriers; emotional barrier; emotional disorders; Emotional disturbances	情感障碍；情绪失调；情绪困扰；情志障碍
endoplasmic reticulum stress-the unfolded protein response pathway; ER stress-UPR pathway	内质网应激——未折叠蛋白反应途径
Endothelial dysfunction; endothelium dysfunction; blood vessel endothelial dysfunction; vascular endothelial dysfunction; endothelial cell dysfunction	内皮功能障碍；内皮功能紊乱；内皮细胞功能障碍；内皮功能不全；内皮功能失调；血管内皮功能障碍；内皮功能损伤；内皮细胞功能紊乱
Endothelin 1; Preproendothelin	血浆内皮素1(ET-1)
Endovascular Interventions; Endovascular treatment; Endovascular therapy; EVT	血管内介入治疗
Energy deficit; Energy depletion; Energy failure	能量耗竭；能量不足；能量耗尽；能量代谢衰竭
enhancing the muscle exercise; Muscle strength training; Strengthening the muscle exercise	增强肌力训练；肌力增强训练
Enlimomab	恩莫单抗
Environmental support assessment; assessment of environmental support; assessment of environment supporting; Evaluation of environment supporting; Evaluation of environmental support	环境支持评价；环境支持度评价；环境支持评估
Ephedrine; ephedrine	麻黄碱；麻黄素
Epidural bleeding; Epidural hemorrhage; Epidural haemorrhage; Epidural haematoma; Epidural hematoma; Epidural intracranial hemorrhage; Epidural intracranial haemorrhage; Epidural intracranial hemorrhage (disorder); Epidural hemorrhage (disorder)	硬膜外出血；硬脑膜外出血；脊柱硬膜外出血
Epilepsy; epilepsy; epilepsia	癫痫；癫痫；癫痫病
Epileptic seizure; seizure; attack; Seizure; Post stroke seizure; Seizure disorder; Seizure disorder (disorder); Epileptic convulsion; Epileptic attack; Epileptic fit; Epileptic seizure (finding)	癫痫发作；癫痫性惊厥
Episodic ataxia; Episodic ataxia (disorder)	发作性共济失调；偶尔发生的共济失调
Episodic quadriplegia; Paroxysmal quadriplegia	阵发性全瘫；发作性四肢瘫痪
Episodic vomiting; Paroxysmal vomiting; paroxysm vomiting	阵发性呕吐；发作性呕吐；间隔性呕吐

续　表

英文术语	中文术语
Erythroblastosis virus E26 oncogene homolog 2; ets-2	成红细胞增多症病毒E26癌基因同源物2
Erythrocyte sedimentation rate; ESR; Erythrocyte sedimentation rate - finding	红细胞沉降率；血沉速率；红细胞沉降速率
Essential mixed cryoglobulinemia; essential mixed cryoglobuline-mia; Essential mixed cryoglobulinemic vasculitis; Essential mixed cryo-globulinaemia; Essential cryoglobulinaemic vasculitis; Essential mixed cryoglobulinemia (disorder)	原发性混合型冷球蛋白血症；原发性混合型冷球蛋白血症性血管炎；紫癜-关节痛-冷球蛋白血症综合征；特发性混合性冷球蛋白血症；特发性混合型冷沉淀球蛋白血症；特发性混合型冷球蛋白血症
Estrogen replacement therapy; Postmenopausal Hormone Replacement Therapy; Estrogen replacement therapies; ERT	雌激素替代治疗；雌激素替代疗法；雌激素替代；雌激素补充疗法；雌激素疗法；雌激素代替疗法
Euphoria; euphoria; Euphoria (finding)	欣快；精神愉快；欣快感；心情愉快症
Evaluation of Atherosclerotic Cerebrovascular Disease; Diagnostic evaluation of Atherosclerotic Cerebrovascular Disease; Atherosclerotic cerebrovascular disease evaluation	动脉粥样硬化性脑血管病评价；动脉粥样硬化性脑血管病的评估；动脉粥样硬化性脑血管病的评价
Evaluation of atherosclerotic cerebrovascular disease risk factors; assessment of atherosclerotic cerebrovascular disease risk factors	动脉粥样硬化性脑血管病危险因素评价；动脉粥样硬化性脑血管病危险因素评估
Evaluation of complications; assessment of complications	并发症评价；并发症评估
Evaluation of Consciousness and Cognitive Function; Evaluation of Consciousness and cognitive evaluation; Evaluation of awareness and cognitive evaluation; Evaluation of awareness and Cognitive Function	意识和认知功能评价
Evaluation table of clinical neurological deficit in stroke patients	脑卒中患者临床神经功能缺损程度评定表；脑卒中患者临床神经功能缺损程度评价表；脑卒中患者临床神经功能缺损程度评分标准
everyday communication needs assessment; Daily communication needs assessment	每日交往需求评价；日常沟通需要评估；日常沟通需要评定
Except stable angina pectoris	除外稳定型心绞痛

续 表

英文术语	中文术语
Excitotoxicity; excitatory toxicity; exitotoxicity; excitotoxic; excitability toxicity; neurotoxicity	兴奋性细胞毒作用；兴奋毒性；兴奋毒；兴奋性毒；兴奋毒作用；兴奋毒损伤；兴奋性毒性损伤；兴奋性毒性
executive impairment; executive function disorders; execution function; Executive dysfunction	执行功能障碍；执行障碍
External carotid artery; External carotid arteries; ECAs; ECA; arteria carotis externa; external carotid artery	颈外动脉
Extracranial to intracranial bypass surgery; EC-IC	行颅内外至颅内旁路手术；颅外 - 颅内搭桥手术
Extrapyramidal dyskinesia; Extrapyramidal motor disorders	锥体外系运动障碍；锥体外系异动症
extrinsic apoptotic pathway	外源性凋亡通路；外在凋亡途径；内源性信号途径
Extrinsic pathway	外源途径；外源性途径 ；外在途径；外凋亡途径
Eyelid apraxia; Apraxia of eyelid; Apraxia of eyelid (disorder)	眼睑失用症；眼皮运用失能症
Ezetimibe	依替米贝；依则替米贝；依哲麦布
F2 isoprostanes; F2IPs; F2IP	F2异前列腺素
Fabry disease; Fabry's disease; Angiokeratoma corporis diffusum universale; Anderson-Fabry disease; GLA deficiency; alpha-Galactosidase-A deficiency; Alpha-galactosidase A deficiency; Fabry's disease (disorder)	法布里病；Fabry's 病；α-半乳糖苷酶缺乏症；法布里病(酰基鞘氨醇己三糖苷酶缺乏症)；法布里氏病；法布里(安德森)病；Fabry-Anderson病；α-半乳糖苷酶-A缺乏；α-半乳糖苷酶A缺乏病；安德森-法布里病；Anderson-Fabry病；α-半乳糖苷酶A缺乏症；α-半乳糖苷酶-A缺乏症；α半乳糖苷酶A缺乏症；Fabry病；法布里(-安德森)病；血管角质瘤综合征；Anderson-Fabry综合征
Facial colliculus syndrome	面丘综合征
Facial paralysis; facial nerve paralysis; Facial nerve paralysis; facial palsy; facial paralysis; Facial palsy; Facial weakness; Facial paresis; Facial palsy (disorder)	面瘫；面神经麻痹；面部神经麻痹；面神经轻瘫；面神经麻痹(面瘫)；面神经瘫
Facial thermoalgesic deficit; Facial thermal hypoesthesia; Facial thermal pain loss	面部痛温觉减退；面部热痛觉缺陷；面部热痛觉缺失

续 表

英文术语	中文术语
Faciobranchial paresis	面臂轻瘫
Factor V Leiden Measurement	因子 V leidon 突变检测
Factor V Leiden mutation; Factor 5 Leiden mutation; Factor V Leiden mutation (disorder)	V 因子 Leiden 突变；莱顿突变；因子 V 莱顿突变
Factor Ⅶ; Coagulation factor Ⅶ	凝血因子Ⅶ；因子Ⅶ
Factor Ⅻ; Coagulation Factor Ⅻ	凝血因子Ⅻ；因子Ⅻ
Familial atrial myxomas; Family atrial myxoma	家族性心房黏液瘤；家族性心房粘液瘤
Familial Combined Hyperlipidemias; Multiple Lipoprotein-Type Hyperlipidemia; Familial Combined Hyperlipidemia	家族性高胆固醇血症；家族性高脂血症；复合脂蛋白型高脂血症
Familial hemiplegic migraine; Familial hemiplegic migraine (disorder); familial hemiplegic migraine; Familial Hemiplegic Migraine	家族性偏瘫型偏头痛；遗传的偏瘫性偏头痛；家族偏瘫性偏头痛；家族性偏瘫性偏头痛
Familial hypertriglyceridemia; familial hypertriglyceridemia; Familial hypertriglyceridaemia; Familial hypertriglyceridemia (disorder)	家族性高甘油三脂血症；家族性高甘油三酯血症；家族性高甘油三酯血症
Familial hypoalphalipoproteinemia; familial hypoalphalipoproteinemia; Hypoalphalipoproteinaemia; hypo α lipoproteinemia; tangier disease; Tangier disease; HDL Lipoprotein Deficiency Disease; Familial HDL deficiency, Type I; HDL Cholesterol, Low Serum; Hypoalphalipoproteinemias; Hypoalphalipoproteinemia; Analphalipoproteinemia; Familial hypoalphalipoproteinaemia; Familial HDL deficiency; Familial high density lipoprotein deficiency; Analphaliproteinaemia; Analphaliproteinemia; Analphalipoproteinaemia; Familial hypoalphalipoproteinemia (disorder); Hypoalphalipoproteinemia (disorder)	家族性低α脂蛋白血病；低α脂蛋白血症；低α-脂蛋白血症；丹吉尔病；Tangier病；家族性高密度脂蛋白缺乏病；家族性HDL缺乏；无α脂蛋白血症；α-脂蛋白缺乏综合征；家族性高密度脂蛋白缺乏症；遗传性高密度脂蛋白缺乏
Family education; home education; family teaching; domestic education	家庭教育；家教；家族教育；家庭教养方式；亲情教育
Family history of stroke; Family history of CVA; family history of stroke	卒中家族史；脑卒中家族史
family support	家庭支持；家庭支持度；家庭养老；家庭帮扶；家属支持；家庭赡养
Fatty acid binding protein; Fatty acid binding proteins; FABPs; FABP	脂肪酸结合蛋白质

英文术语	中文术语
Fatty meats; Fatty meat	肥肉；白肉
Favorable outcome; Good outcomes	预后良好；结局良好；疗效良好
Feeding test	进食试验；喂养实验；试食试验；喂养试验
Fiber intake; Dietary fibre intake	纤维摄入；纤维素摄入；纤维摄入量
Fiber optic endoscopy swallowing assessment	纤维光学内镜吞咽评估；纤维内镜吞咽评估
Fibrates; Fibric acid derivatives; Fibrate	贝特类
Fibrillation; fibrillation; Fibrillation (disorder); ventricular fibrillation	肌纤维震颤；心室颤动
Fibrin; fibrin	纤维蛋白；血纤蛋白
Fibrinogen; Coagulation factor I; Factor I; fibrinogen	纤维蛋白原；血纤蛋白原
Fibrinopeptide A; FPA	血纤维蛋白肽A
Fibromuscular dysplasia; FMD; fibromuscular dysplasia	肌纤维发育不良；纤维肌性发育不良；纤维肌发育不良
Fibromuscular dysplasia of carotid artery; Carotid fibromuscular dysplasia	颈动脉纤维肌发育不良；颈动脉纤维异常增生；颈动脉肌纤维发育不良
Fibromuscular dysplasia of renal artery; Fibromuscular hyperplasia of renal artery; FMH - Fibromuscular hyperplasia, of renal artery	肾动脉纤维肌性发育不良；肾动脉肌纤维发育不良
Finger agnosia; Finger agnosia (finding)	手指失认；手指失认症
finger skin temperature biofeedback therapy; FSTBFT	手指温度生物反馈疗法
Fish intake; Fish consumption; Fish; fish	鱼；鱼类
Fish oil; Fish oils; anchovy oil; dace oil; omega 3 fish oil; fish oil aprico; marine fish oil	鱼油；鱼油脂肪乳；淡水鱼油；鱼油油脂；鱼肝油
FLAIR weighted images; Fluid attenuated inversion recovery-weighted imaging; FLAIR-weighted images	FLAIR加权图像
Flavonoids; Bioflavonoids; Flavonoid; flavanoids; flavanoid; flavonols	黄酮类；黄酮；类黄酮；黄酮类物质
fluorodeoxyglucose positron emission tomography; fluorodeoxy-glucose PET	氟脱氧葡萄糖正电子发射断层成像；氟脱氧葡萄糖正电子发射断层扫描术

续 表

英文术语	中文术语
Focal dystonia; focal dystonia; Focal dystonia (disorder)	局限性肌张力障碍；灶性张力障碍；局灶型肌张力障碍
Folic acid intake; Folate intake	叶酸摄入
Forced grasping reflex; grasp reflex; Grasp reflex	握持反射；强握反射
Foville syndrome; Inferior medial pontine syndrome; foville syndrome; Foville syndrome (disorder)	Foville综合征；福维尔综合征；Foville氏综合征
free fatty acid	游离脂肪酸
Free radical synthesis; Free radical generation; Free radical formation; Free radicals; Free radical	自由基合成；自由基；自由基形成；自由基生成
Frenchay Activities Index; FAI	Frenchay活动量表
Frenchay activity index	Frenchay活动指数
Frenchay Aphasia Screening Test; FAST	Frenchay构音障碍评价法
Fried food intake; Fried food taking	油炸食物摄入量；油炸食品摄入
Frontal brain region	额叶脑区
Frontoparietal brain region	额顶脑区
Frontotemporal brain region	额颞部脑区
Fruit; Consumption of fruits; Consumption of fruit; Fruits	水果；果实
Fugl Meyer Assessment; Fugl-Meyer Assessment of Sensorimotor Recovery After Stroke; FM assessment; FMA; Fugl-Myer Scale	Fugl-Meyer评定法
function evaluation; functional evaluation; functional assessment; functional estimate; functions evaluation; function valuation; functional appraisal	功能评价；功能评估
function impairment; functional deficit; functional defect; function deficiency; function deficit; function damage; functional defects; functional deficiency	功能缺陷；功能损害；功能缺损
Functional Ambulation Category; Functional Ambulation Categories; FAC; Functional Ambulation Classification	功能性步行量表
functional communication profile; FCP	功能性交际测验
functional communication therapy; FCT	功能性交际治疗
Functional comorbidity index; FCI	功能性共病指数

英文术语	中文术语
functional electrical stimulation therapy; fonctional electrical stimulation; functional electrical stimulation; FES	功能性电刺激疗法
Functional Indenpendence Measure; Functional independence assessment; function independent measure; FIM	功能独立性评定(FIM)；功能独立评测量表；功能独立性测评量表
functional reach test	功能性及物试验；功能前伸试验；功能性前伸测试；功能性前伸试验；功能伸展测试
Furosemide; furosemide	呋塞米；速尿
gait; gaits; gait patterns; gait pattern; walking gait	步态；步姿；步法
Gait apraxia; Apraxia of gait; Apraxic gait; Gait apraxia (finding)	步态失用；步态失调
Gait ataxia; Ataxic gait; Tabetic gait; Ataxic gait (finding)	共济失调步态；步态共济失调；共济失调性步态；脊髓痨步态
galvanic skin response biofeedback therapy; GSRBFT	直流电皮肤反应生物反馈疗法；皮肤电阻生物反馈疗法
Gamma aminobutyrate; Increase of Gamma aminobutyrate	γ氨基丁酸酯；γ-氨基丁酸；γ氨基丁酸酯增加
gamma Aminobutyric acid agonist; GABA Receptor Agonist	γ氨基丁酸激动剂
Gastritis; gastritis; Gastritis (disorder)	胃炎
Gastrointestinal bleeding; GI bleeding; GIB; gastrointestinal bleeding; gastrointestinal hemorrhage; Gastrointestinal Hemorrhage; Gastrointestinal hemorrhage; Gastrointestinal haemorrhage; GI - Gastrointestinal bleed; GI - Gastrointestinal haemorrhage; GI - Gastrointestinal hemorrhage; GIT - Gastrointestinal tract haemorrhage; GIT - Gastrointestinal tract hemorrhage; Gastrointestinal bleed; GIH - Gastrointestinal haemorrhage; GIH - Gastrointestinal hemorrhage; GI haemorrhage; GI hemorrhage; Gastrointestinal hemorrhage (disorder)	消化道出血；胃肠出血；GI 出血
gatism; Bowel and Bladder Incontinence; incontinence	尿便障碍；大小便失禁
Gaze-evoked horizontal nystagmus; Gazeevoked horizontal nystagmus	凝视诱发性水平眼震；凝视性眼震；凝视诱发水平眼球震颤
Gaze-evoked nystagmus; Gazeevoked nystagmus	凝视诱发性眼球震颤；凝视诱发眼震；凝视性眼震；凝视诱发性眼震

续　表

英文术语	中文术语
Gemfibrozil	吉非贝齐；优瑞脂；洁脂；乐衡吉非罗齐
Gender; sex factors; Patient sex; sex factor; Sex	性别；性交行为；性别因素
Gene expression; genes expression; genetic expression; gene express; gene; gene expressions; gene expressed; gene expressing; Gene response	基因表达；早期基因反应；基因应答；基因反应
General treatment; general therapy	一般疗法；一般治疗
Generalized dystonia; generalized dystonia; Generalised dystonia; Generalized dystonia (disorder)	全身型肌张力障碍；泛发性张力失常；全面性肌张力障碍
Genes that control serum bilirubin	控制血清胆红素的基因
Genetic risk factor; Heredity risk factor; Genetic risk factors; Genetics risk factor; Heredity factors; Genetic factors; Heredity factor; Genetic factor; Genetic	遗传因素；遗传危险因素；共同危险因素；基因风险因子
Genomic biomarkers of hemorrhagic stroke	出血性脑卒中的基因组生物标志物
Genomics biomarkers of stroke	脑卒中的基因组学生物标志物
Geographic area; geographic factors; geographic factor	地区；地理；地理区域
Gerstmann syndrome; Angular gyrus syndrome; gerstmann syndrome; Gerstmann's syndrome	Gerstmann综合征；格斯特曼综合征；格斯特曼综合症
Glasgow Coma Scale; GCS	格拉斯哥昏迷评分；格拉斯哥昏迷量表；格拉斯哥昏迷量表评分；Glasgow昏迷量表
Glasgow Outcome Scale; GOS	格拉斯哥结局量表；格拉斯哥结果分级；格拉斯哥预后量表；GOS量表；Glasgow预后评价；Glasgow预后评分
Glaucomatous visual field defect; Glaucomatous visual field defect (finding)	青光眼性视野缺损；青光眼视野缺损
Glia biomarkers of stroke; Glia biomarker of stroke	脑卒中胶质生物标志物
Glial fibrillary acidic protein; Glial fibrillary-associated protein; GFAP	胶质纤维酸性蛋白
glucose control; Blood sugar control; Blood glucose control; glycemic control; blood glucose; metabolic control; glycaemic control; blood glucose controlling	控制血糖；血糖调控

英文术语	中文术语
glucosylceramide; GlcCer	葡糖神经酰胺
GluN1; l-glutamic acid; l-glutamate	谷氨酸 1
glutamate; glutamic acid; Glutamic acid; Increase of glutamate	谷氨酸；谷氨酸增加；谷氨酸盐；谷氨酸酯
Glutamate binds to N methyl D aspartate receptor; Binding of glutamic acid to N methyl D aspartate receptor; Glutamate binds to NMDA receptor	谷氨酸与 N- 甲基 -D- 天冬氨酸受体结合
Glutamate excitotoxicity; Glutamate release	谷氨酸兴奋性毒性；谷氨酸释放
Glutathione; glutathione; glutathion; GSH	谷胱甘肽；谷胱苷肽；谷光甘肽
Glutathione S transferase P	谷胱甘肽 S 转移酶 P
Glycemic control; blood glucose control; glycemic control; glucose control; blood glucose; metabolic control; glycaemic control; blood sugar control	血糖控制；血糖控制状态；控制血糖；血糖调控；血糖水平控制；血糖控制水平
Glycerol; Glycerine; glycerol	甘油；甘油糖原
glycerophosphoethanolamine	磷脂酰乙醇胺
glycine; Glycine; Increase of glycine	甘氨酸；甘油酸；氨基醋酸；氨基乙酸；甘氨酸增加
glycine antagonist; glycine antagonists; glycine inhibitor	甘氨酸拮抗剂
glycogen phosphorylase	糖原磷酸化酶
Glycomics biomarkers of stroke	脑卒中的糖组学生物标志物
go to the toilet; toilet	如厕；上厕所
good limb position; good limb position placement; good limb display; placement of good limbs; good limb placement; good limb place; healthy limb placement; put a good limb position	良肢位摆放
Grain; Whole grain; Whole-grain; Grains	谷物；粮食；稻谷
Granulomatous angitis of central nervous system; primary angiitis of central nervous system; Idiopathic angiitis of central nervous system; Primary angiitis of central nervous system (disorder); Primary angiitis of central nervous system; PACNS; Granulomatous angiitis of central nervous system; Granulomatous angiitis of central nervous system (disorder)	中枢神经系统原发性血管炎；中枢神经系统肉芽肿性脉管炎；中枢神经系统肉芽肿性血管炎；原发性中枢神经系统血管炎
Graphomania; scribomania	书写狂；笔墨病

续　表

英文术语	中文术语
Green leafy vegetables; Green leafy vegetable	绿叶蔬菜；绿叶菜；绿叶类蔬菜
group language training	小组语言训练
group therapy; team treatment; group intervention; group treatment; group training	群体治疗；团体辅导；团体疗法；集体治疗；集体疗法；团体治疗；小组治疗
Guiding airflow method; steering flow method	引导气流法；转向流量法
Hallucinations; hallucination; Hallucination; hallucinations; Illusions; Illusion; Illusions (finding); Hallucinations (finding)	幻觉
Hamartomatous tumor syndrome	错构瘤性肿瘤综合征；哈马瘤样肿瘤综合征；错构瘤综合征
Hamilton Depression Scale; HAMD	汉密顿抑郁量表；汉密尔顿抑郁评分；哈密顿抑郁量表；汉密顿抑郁量表评分；HAMD抑郁量表；Hamilton抑郁量表
Hamrin activity index	Hamrin活动指数
Hand muscle strength; Hand muscle force; Hand muscle forces; Hand muscle ability	手肌力；手部肌肉力量
Hand tremor; Hands tremor	手部震颤；手震颤
Haptoglobin; HP	结合珠蛋白
Head deviation; Head deflection; Head deflect; Head skew	头偏转；头偏；头部偏斜
Head tremor; head tremor	头部震颤；头震颤
Headache; headache; Head Pain; Cephalgia; Cephalalgia; Cephalodynia; Head pain; Pain in head; HA - Headache; Headache (finding); Headache disorder; Headache disorder (disorder)	头痛；头痛病；头疼；头部疼痛；头痛或头疼
Headache (with pheochromocytoma)	头痛(伴嗜铬细胞瘤)；头痛（伴发嗜铬细胞瘤）
health education; healthy education; heath education; healthy educational; health care education; idd health education; athletics education	健康教育；健康宣教；卫生教育；健康教育学；卫生宣教；宣传教育；健康教育方法；健康教育指导
hearing; auditory; auditory event; audition; sense of hearing; auditory sense	听觉；听力

英文术语	中文术语
Hearing impairment; hard-of-hearing; Hearing worse; deafness; Anacusis; Deafness; Hearing impaired; HI - Hearing impairment; HL - Hearing loss; HOH - Hard of hearing; Hard of hearing; Hearing difficulty; Hearing difficulty (finding); Hearing worse (finding)	听觉减退；耳聋；听力损伤；听力损害；听觉损失；听力损失；听力缺损；听力丧失；听力受损；听觉受损；听力减退；听觉丧失；听力障碍
Heart failure; heart failure; Heart Failure; cardiac failure; heartfailure; Cardiac insufficiency; Cardiac failure; HF - Heart failure; Myocardial failure; Heart failure (disorder); Congestive heart failure	心力衰竭；心脏功能不全；心脏衰弱；心衰；充血性心力衰竭
heart rate bio-feedback therapy; HRBFT	心率生物反馈疗法
Heart type fatty acid binding protein; H-FABP; HFABP	心脏型脂肪酸结合蛋白
heat therapy; thermotherapy	热疗法；温热疗法
heavy drinking; Binge alcohol drinking; Heavy alcohol consumption; Drinking binge; Binge drinking; Alcohol abuse; Alcohol binge; Alcohol; alcohol; Ethanol abuse; Ethanol; alcohol abuse; ALCOHOL ABUSE; binge drinking; Drinking binge (finding); AA - Alcohol abuse; Alcohol abuse (disorder)	酗酒；酒精；酒精滥用；狂饮；狂饮性饮酒
Hematologic Tests; Blood routine test; Blood tests; blood detection; blood routine testing	血液检测；血液检查；血常规；血常规检验；血常规检查
Hemianacusia; single-sided deafness	单侧聋；偏侧聋；一侧聋
Hemianopia; hemianopia; hemianopsia; Hemianopia (finding); Hemianopsia	偏盲；一侧视力缺失
Hemiataxia	偏身共济失调；偏身运动失调；偏失动症
Hemiballismus; hemiballismus; Hemiballismus-hemichorea syndrome; Hemiballism (disorder); Hemichorea hemiballismus; Hemiballism	单侧抽搐；偏身颤抽；偏身抽搐
Hemifacial anhydrosis; Sudomotor dysfunction; Hemifacial anhidrosis; Sweating dysfunction; Lack of sweating	偏侧面部无汗；泌汗功能异常
Hemifacial spasm; Spasticity of facial muscles; Facial spasm; Hemifacial Spasm; hemifacial spasm; facial spasm; hemi-facial spasm; Hemifacial spasm (finding); Facial spasm (finding)	偏侧面肌痉挛；面部单侧痉挛；偏侧颜面痉挛；偏侧面肌痉挛症；面肌痉挛；面痉挛；面部痉挛

续 表

英文术语	中文术语
Hemihypesthesia; hemianesthesia; Hemihypesthesia with cognitive disturbance; Hemihypoesthesia; Hemihypaesthesia; Hemianesthesia; Hemianaesthesia; Hemisensory loss; Hemianesthesia (finding)	偏身感觉减退；偏侧感觉缺失；半身麻木；偏身麻木
hemihypoesthesia without cognitive impairment; hemihypoesthesia without cognition disorders; hemihypoesthesia without cognitive dysfunction; Hemihypesthesia without cognitive disturbance	无认知障碍的偏身感觉减退；偏身感觉迟钝无认知障碍；没有认知障碍的偏身感觉迟钝
Hemihypokinesia; hypokinetic disease	少动症；运动不足病
Hemimedullary infarction symptom; Babinski Nageotte syndrome	延髓半侧综合征；延髓半侧梗死症状
Hemineglect; Hemispatial Neglect; Unilateral neglect; Hemineglect; Hemiagnosia; Hemi-neglect (finding)	偏侧忽略；单方面忽略
Hemiparesis; hemiparesis; HEMIPARESIS; Hemiparesis (weakness on one side); Hemiparesis (disorder)	轻偏瘫；轻度偏瘫
Hemiplegic Shoulder Pain; post-stroke shoulder pain	偏瘫肩痛；偏瘫肩痛患者；卒中后肩痛；偏瘫性肩痛
Hemispheric infarction syndrome; syndromes of hemispheric infarction; syndrome of hemispheric infarction; Hemispheric infarction syndromes; Hemispheric infarction symptoms; Hemispheric infarction symptom	大脑半球梗死综合征
Hemispheric Stroke Scale	半球卒中量表；半球脑卒中评定量表
Hemoglobin concentration; Haemoglobin concentration	血红蛋白浓度；平均血红蛋白含量；血红蛋白含量
Hemorrhagic stroke	出血性卒中
Hemorrhagic transformation	出血转化
Hemostatic biomarkers of stroke; Hemostatic biomarker of stroke	脑卒中的止血生物标志物
Hemostatic factors; Hemostatic factor; Haemostatic factors; Haemostatic factor	止血因素；止血因子
Henoch-schonlein purpura	过敏性紫癜；反复发作过敏性紫癜；Henoch-schonlein紫癜；亨-舍二氏紫癜
Heparin; heparin; calparine	肝素；肝磷脂；肝制凝素
Hereditary cardiac conduction disorder; Hereditary cardiac conduction disorders	遗传性心脏传导障碍

英文术语	中文术语
Hereditary cardiomyopathy; genetic cardiomyopathy; inherited cardiomyopathy	遗传性心肌病
Hereditary dyslipoproteinemia; Hereditary dyslipoproteinemias	遗传性脂蛋白血症
Hereditary hemorrhagic telangiectasia; Osler hemorrhagic telangiectasia syndrome; Osler-Weber-Rendu disease; Rendu-Weber disease; HHT; Osler haemorrhagic telangiectasia syndrome; Osler's disease; HHT - Hereditary haemorrhagic telangiectasia; HHT - Hereditary hemorrhagic telangiectasia; Hereditary haemorrhagic telangiectasia; Osler-Rendu-Weber disease; Osler-Rendu-Weber syndrome; Osler hemorrhagic telangiectasia syndrome (disorder)	遗传性出血性毛细血管扩张症；奥斯勒出血性毛细血管扩张综合症；遗传性毛细血管扩张症；奥斯勒-韦伯-朗迪病；Osler 病；奥斯勒氏病；奥斯勒病；Osler 出血性毛细血管扩张综合征；遗传性出血性毛细血管扩张；郎-奥韦综合征；Babington 病；Osler-Rendu-Weber 综合征；Goldstein 综合征；遗传性出血性毛细管扩张；Rendu-Osler-Weber 病；奥-朗-韦三氏综合征；奥斯勒出血性毛细血管扩张综合征；Osler-Weber-Rendu 病；奥斯勒-韦伯-朗迪综合征；韦伯三氏病
Hereditary hemorrhagic telangiectasia type 1; HHT1; hereditary hemorrhagic telangiectasis type 1; hereditary haemorrhagic telangiectasia type 1	遗传性出血性毛细血管扩张症 1 型；1 型遗传性出血性毛细血管扩张；遗传出血性毛细血管扩张 1 型；遗传性出血性毛细血管扩张 1 型；1 型遗传性出血性毛细血管扩张症；遗传性毛细血管扩张症 1 型；遗传性、出血性毛细血管扩张症 1 型
Hereditary hemorrhagic telangiectasia type 2; hereditary hemorrhagic telangiectasis type 2; hereditary haemorrhagic telangiectasia type 2; HHT2	遗传性出血性毛细血管扩张症 2 型；遗传性、出血性毛细血管扩张症 2 型；2 型遗传性出血性毛细血管扩张；遗传出血性毛细血管扩张 2 型；遗传性出血性毛细血管扩张 2 型；2 型遗传性出血性毛细血管扩张症；遗传性毛细血管扩张症 2 型

英文术语	中文术语
Hereditary hemorrhagic telangiectasia type 3; HHT3; hereditary hemorrhagic telangiectasis type 3; hereditary haemorrhagic telangiectasia type 3	遗传性出血性毛细血管扩张症3型；3型遗传性出血性毛细血管扩张；遗传出血性毛细血管扩张3型；遗传性出血性毛细血管扩张3型；3型遗传性出血性毛细血管扩张症；遗传性毛细血管扩张症3型；遗传性、出血性毛细血管扩张症3型
Hereditary hemorrhagic telangiectasia type 4; HHT4; hereditary hemorrhagic telangiectasis type 4; hereditary haemorrhagic telangiectasia type 4	遗传性出血性毛细血管扩张症4型；4型遗传性出血性毛细血管扩张；遗传出血性毛细血管扩张4型；遗传性出血性毛细血管扩张4型；4型遗传性出血性毛细血管扩张症；遗传性毛细血管扩张症4型；遗传性、出血性毛细血管扩张症4型
Heroin; heroin	海洛因；二乙酰吗啡
Heteronymous hemianopia; heteronymous hemianopsia; Heteronymous hemianopsia; Heteronymous hemianopsia (finding)	对侧偏盲；交叉偏盲
hexokinase 2; HK2	己糖激酶2
Hiccups; hiccup; Hiccoughs; Hiccup; Singultus; Observation of hiccoughs; Finding of hiccoughs; Hiccoughs (finding); Hiccough	呃逆；打呃；呃逆病；呃逆症
High alpha linolenic acid intake; High alpha-linolenic acid diet intake	高α-亚麻酸摄入量
High density lipoprotein; High-density lipoprotein; Good cholesterol; HDL	高密度脂蛋白
High intracranial pressure; intracranial hypertension; Increased intracranial pressure; Raised intracranial pressure; Increased ICP; High ICP; Increased intracranial pressure; RIP - Raised intracranial pressure; Raised intracranial pressure (finding)	颅内压增高；颅内高压；颅内压升高；颅内压增加；颅内压力增高
High magnesium intake; magnesium intake; magnesium	高镁摄入量；镁；镁离子
High n-3 polyunsaturated fatty acid diet; Plant-derived omega-3 (n-3) polyunsaturated fatty acids; Fish oils drived omega 3 polyunsaturated fatty acids; Omega 3 polyunsaturated fatty acids; Omega 3 polyunsaturated fatty acid; Omega 3 fatty acids	高n-3多不饱和脂肪酸饮食
High n-6 polyunsaturated fatty acid diet	高n-6多不饱和脂肪酸饮食

续　表

英文术语	中文术语
High potassium intake; potassium intake; Potassium; potassium	高钾饮食；钾素；钾离子
High protein intake; High protein food; High protein diet; Increased protein diet; HP - High protein diet; HPD - High protein diet; Increased protein diet (finding)	高蛋白饮食
High-density lipoprotein cholesterol; high density lipoprotein cholesterol; HDL-C; HDLC	高密度脂蛋白胆固醇(HDL-C)
Hippocampus; hippocampus	海马；海马脑区
Histological biomarkers of stroke	脑卒中的组织学生物标志物
History of Bleeding; hemorrhage history; bleeding history	出血史
History of medications; medication history; History of drug; drug history	用药史
History of myocardial infarction	心肌梗死病史
History of Stroke; History of stroke in last year	既往卒中史
History of Surgery; operation history; operative history; previous surgery; previous surgical history	手术史
History of Transient ischemic attack; Previous transient ischemic attack; History of TIAs; History of TIA; Previous TIA	短暂性脑缺血发作史
History of Trauma; traumatic history; injury history; trauma history	外伤史；创伤史
Hoarseness; Hoarse; hoarseness; Hoarse voice; Hoarse voice quality; Hoarseness - throat symptom; Hoarseness symptom; Voice hoarseness; Hoarse (finding)	声音嘶哑；声嘶的；声嘶；声哑；嘶哑
Home Healthcare Agency; HHCA; Family health care institutions; family health nursing institutions; home health care institutions; Family health care organization; family health nursing organization; home health care organization; Family health care agencies; family health nursing agencies; home health care agencies	家庭健康护理机构；家庭卫生保健机构
homocysteine metabolic pathway; Hcy metabolism	同型半胱氨酸代谢途径
Homocystinuria; hypercystinuria; homocystinuria; Homocystinuria (disorder); Deficiency of serine sulphydrase; Cystathionine beta-synthase deficiency (disorder); Cystathionine beta-synthase deficiency; CBS deficiency; Deficiency of beta-thionase; Deficiency of methylcysteine synthase; Deficiency of serine sulfhydrase	高胱氨酸尿症；同型胱氨酸尿症；假性Marfan综合征；高胱氨酸尿；胱硫醚β-合酶缺乏；CBS缺乏；CBS缺乏症；胱硫醚β-合酶缺乏症；胱硫醚β-合酶乏；胱硫醚β合成酶缺乏症
Homolateral ataxia; ipsilateral ataxia	同侧共济失调；同侧运动失调

续　表

英文术语	中文术语
Homonymous hemianopia; homonymous hemianopsia; Homonymous hemianopsia; Homonymous bilateral visual field defects; HH - Homonymous hemianopia; Homonymous hemianopia (finding)	同向性偏盲；同侧偏盲；同侧性双侧视野缺损
Homonymous quadrantanopsia; homonomous quadrantanopsia	同侧象限盲；同侧象限性盲
Horizontal conjugate gaze palsy	水平共轭注视麻痹
Horizontal gaze; horizon gaze; horizon gazing; Horizontal gazing; Horizontal visual	水平凝视；横向凝视；水平注视
Horizontal gaze paresis; Lateral gaze paralysis	水平凝视麻痹；水平侧视麻痹；水平注视麻痹
Horizontal ipsilateral gaze palsy	水平同侧注视麻痹
Horizontal jerk nystagmus; Horizontal acute nystagmus	水平跳动性眼球震颤；水平突起性眼震；水平跳动性眼震
Horizontal nystagmus; horizontal nystagmus; Horizontal nystagmus (disorder)	水平性眼震；水平性眼球震颤；水平眼震
horizontal optokinetic nystagmus; Horizontal opticokinetic nystagmus	水平性视动性眼球震颤；水平视动性眼震
Horizontal pendular nystagmus; Transverse swinging eyeball tremor; Transverse swinging ocular tremor	水平钟摆性眼球震颤；水平坠状眼球震颤
horizontal sectoranopias	水平扇形偏盲；水平扇形弱视
Horner syndrome; Ipsilateral Horner syndrome; Oculosympathetic palsy; horner syndrome; Horner's syndrome	霍纳综合征；Horner 综合征；Horner 综合征；小儿颈交感神经麻痹综合征；颈交感神经麻痹(霍纳氏综合征)；Bernard-Horner综合征；Claude-Bernard-Horner综合征；颈交感神经麻痹综合征
household; domestic affairs; household affairs; housework; domesticity	家务；内部事务；家事
Hufschmidt therapy; Spastic electrical stimulation therapy; Spastic electrical stimulating therapy; Spastic electric stimulating therapy; Spastic electrostimulation therapy	痉挛肌电刺激疗法
Hunt and hess scale	Hunt-Hess 分级
Hydrostatic pad; static pressure pad; static pressure cushion; static pressure pads; static pressure flotation cushion	液压垫；静压垫；静态压力垫

续　表

英文术语	中文术语
Hydroxyl radicals; Hydroxyl; OH	羟基自由基；羟基
hydroxylase; Increase of hydroxylase	羟化酶；羟基化酶；酪胺 -β 羟化酶；羟化酶增加；羟化酶类；苯酚羟化酶
Hypercholesteremia; High Cholesterol Level; Hypercholesterolemias; Elevated Cholesterols; Hypercholesterolemia; Elevated cholesterol; Hypercholesteremias; Hypercholesterolaemia; Hypercholesterolemia (disorder)	高胆固醇血症；高胆固醇
Hyperfibrinogenemia; Elevated plasma fibrinogen; Increased fibrinogen; Hyperfibrinogenaemia; Hyperfibrinogenemia (disorder)	高纤维蛋白原血症；血纤维蛋白原过多症
Hyperglycemia; hyperglycemia; Hyperglycaemia; Hyperglycemia (disorder); High blood glucose; High blood sugar; Hyperglycemic disorder; Hyperglycaemic disorder; Hyperglycemic disorder (disorder)	高血糖；高血糖症；高糖血症
Hyperglycemia control	高血糖控制
Hypergraphia	强迫书写
Hyperinsulinemia; hyperinsulinism; Hyperinsulinism; Hyperinsulinaemia; Hyperinsulinism (disorder)	高胰岛素血症；高胰岛素血；超高胰岛素血症
Hyperlipidaemia; HLD - Hyperlipidaemia; HLD - Hyperlipidemia; Lipidaemia; Hyperlipidemia (disorder); Hyperlipidemias; Hyperlipidemia; Hyperlipemias; Hyperlipemia; Lipidemias; Lipidemia; Lipemias; Lipemia	高脂血症；脂血 (症)；高血脂症；脂血症
Hyperlipidemia due to type 2 diabetes mellitus; Hyperlipidaemia due to type 2 diabetes mellitus; Hyperlipidemia due to T2DM; Hyperlipidemia due to type 2 diabetes mellitus (disorder)	2 型糖尿病引起的高脂血症；T2DM 所致高脂血症；T2DM 引起的高脂血症
Hyperlipoproteinemias; Hyperlipoproteinaemia; hyperlipoproteinemia; hyperlipaemia; Hyperlipoproteinemia; Hyperlipoproteinemia (disorder)	高脂蛋白血症；高蛋白血症
Hyperphosphorylated tau protein	过度磷酸化 tau 蛋白

续　表

英文术语	中文术语
Hypersensitivity vasculitis; Cutaneous vasculitis; Leukocytoclastic vasculitis; Leucocytoclastic angiitis; Leukocytoclastic vasculitis; Leukocytoclastic angiitis; Hypersensitivity angiitis (disorder); Hypersensitivity angiitis; Allergic vasculitis; Hypersensitivity vasculitides; hypersensitivity vasculitis	过敏性血管炎；变应性血管炎；白细胞破碎性血管炎；白细胞分裂性脉管炎；白细胞碎裂性血管炎；白细胞分裂性血管炎；超敏反应血管炎；超敏感性血管炎；过敏性脉管炎；超敏性血管炎；白细胞破裂性血管炎；皮肤白细胞破碎性血管炎；皮肤白细胞碎裂性血管炎；变应性脉管炎；变应性小动脉炎；坏死性结节性皮炎；结节性真皮过敏疹
Hypersomnia; Excessive sleep; Excessive sleepiness; Hypersomnia (excessive sleeping); Hypersomnia (disorder); Hypersomnolence	嗜睡；过度睡眠；睡眠过度(多)；睡眠过度；过度嗜睡；睡眠过多
Hypertension; High blood pressure; HTN; hypertension; Essential hypertension; essential hypertension; Primary hypertension; Idiopathic hypertension; Systemic primary arterial hypertension; Essential hypertension (disorder); Hypertensive disorder; Hypertensive disease; Hyperpiesis; Hyperpiesia; BP - High blood pressure; High blood pressure disorder; HBP - High blood pressure; BP+ - Hypertension; HT - Hypertension; HTN - Hypertension	高血压；原发性高血压；原发性高血压病；系统性原发性动脉性高血压；高血压待查；特发性(原发性)高血压；高血压病；高血压症
Hypertonic Saline; hyperosmotic saline; hypertonic salin; saline solution, hypertonic; hypertonic saline water; high permeability brine	高渗盐水；高渗盐溶液；高渗盐液；高张盐溶液；高张氯化钠
Hypertriglyceridemia; Elevated triglycerides; Hypertriglyceridemias; hypertriglyceridemia; Hypertriglyceridaemia; Hypertriglyceridemia (disorder)	高甘油三酯血症；高三酰甘油血症；高甘油三脂血症；高三酸甘油脂血症
Hyperuricemia; hyperuricemia; Hyperuricuria; Hyperuricuria (disorder); Hyperuricaemia; Hyperuricemia (disorder)	高尿酸血症；尿酸血症；高尿酸尿症
Hyperventilation; hyperventilation; overventilation; Hyperventilating; Hyperventilation (finding)	过度换气；换气过度；过度呼吸
Hypervigilance; Hyperarousal	过度警觉；警觉过度
Hyperviscosity; hyperviscosity; Hyperviscosity (finding)	高黏滞血症；高粘血症；高黏血症；高血粘度

英文术语	中文术语
Hypesthesia; hypesthesia; Has numbness; Has numbness (finding); Numbness; Deadness - numbness; Numbness (finding); Hypoaesthesia; Hypoesthesia; Hypoaesthesia (reduced sensation); Hypoesthesia (reduced sensation); Hypesthesia (finding)	麻木；麻木(感)
Hypnagogic hallucinations; Hypnagogic hallucination; Hypnagogic hallucinations (finding)	入睡前幻觉；临睡幻觉；入睡幻觉
Hypnic headache; hypnic headache; Hypnic headache (associated with sleep); Hypnic headache (disorder)	睡眠性头痛
Hypnopompic hallucinations; hypnagogic hallucination	初醒幻觉；催眠幻觉
Hypofibrinogenemia; Hypodysfibrinogenemia; HYPOFIBRINO-GENEMIA; Hypofibrinogenaemia; Hypofibrinogenemia (disorder); Hypodysfibrinogenaemia; Hypodysfibrinogenemia (disorder)	低纤维蛋白原血症；低纤维素原血症；低纤维蛋白血症
Hypoglycemia; hypoglycaemia; Hypoglycemic disorder; Hyperschemazia; Low blood sugar; hypoglycemia; Hypoglycaemic disorder; Hypoglycemic disorder (disorder); Hyperschemazia (disorder); Hypoglycaemia; Hypoglycemia (disorder)	低血糖；血糖偏低；低血糖症；低糖血症；低血糖病；血糖偏低症
Hypoglycemic coma; hypoglycemic coma; Hypoglycaemic coma; Hypoglycemic coma (disorder)	低血糖昏迷；低血糖性昏迷；低血糖性无意识；血糖过低性昏迷
Hypoglycemic control	低血糖症的控制；降血糖控制
Hypolipidaemia; Hypolipidemia; Hypolipidemia (disorder)	低脂血症
hypoperfusion/ impaired emboli clearance; Hypoperfusion; Reduce cerbral blood flow; Reduce CBF	低灌注/栓子清除率下降；低灌注；减少颅内血流量
Hypophonia; Hypophonia (finding)	发音过弱；发声过弱
hypoplasminogenemia; Low fibrinogen	低纤溶酶原血症；低血浆酶原血
Hypotension; Low blood pressure; hypotension; Hypopiesis; Arterial hypotension; Low blood pressure (disorder)	低血压；动脉低血压；低血压症；动脉性低血压
Hypothermia; hypothermia; Hypothermia (finding)	低体温；低体温症
hypoxanthine; Increase of hypoxanthine	次黄嘌呤；6-羟基嘌呤；6-氧嘌呤；次黄瞟呤；次黄嘌呤；黄嘌呤；次黄嘌呤含量增加
Hypoxemia; hypoxemia; hypoxia; Hypoxia; Hypoxemias; Anoxemia; Anoxia; Anoxaemia; Hypoxic; Hypoxia (disorder); Hypoxaemia; Hypoxemia (disorder)	低氧血症；低氧血；低氧；低氧症；低血氧症；低血氧；动脉低氧血

续　表

英文术语	中文术语
hypoxia inducible factor 1 alpha subunit; HIF1A	缺氧诱导因子1α亚基
Ideomotor apraxia; Ideomotor dyspraxia; Ideomotor dyspraxia (disorder)	观念运动性失用；观念运动性失用症
Immune cell therapy	免疫细胞治疗；免疫细胞疗法
Immune mediator; immune amboceptor; Immune mediators	免疫介体；免疫介质
Immune responce; immune responses; immunity response; mediated immune responses; immunoresponse; immunological response; mediated immune response	免疫应答
immune response pathway; immune responses pathway; immunity response pathway; mediated immune responses pathway; immunoresponse pathway; immunological response pathway	免疫应答途径；免疫反应途径
immunomodulatory therapy; Immunomodulatory therapeutic; immunomodulation; immunoloregulation; immune regulation	免疫调节治疗；免疫调节
Impaired glucose tolerance; impaired glucose tolerance; Abnormal glucose tolerance; IGT - Impaired glucose tolerance; Impaired glucose tolerance (disorder); IGT; Abnormal glucose tolerance test; Abnormal glucose tolerance test (finding)	糖耐量异常；糖耐量减低；葡萄糖耐量降低；葡萄糖耐量受损；糖耐量降低；葡萄糖耐量异常
Impulsivity; Impulse; impulsivity; impulse	冲动
Increase of biochemical substances; Increase of chemical substance; Increase of biochemical materials; Increase of biochemical metabolites; Increase of biological compound; Increase of biochemical; Increase in biochemical substances; Increase of biochemical substances; Increase of biochemical substance	生化物质增加
Increased blood viscocity	血液黏稠度增加；血液黏度增加
Indomethacin; Indometacin	吲哚美辛；消炎痛
Inducible nitric oxide synthase; NOS2; iNOS	诱导型一氧化氮合酶；诱生型一氧化氮合酶；诱导性一氧化氮合酶；内皮型一氧化氮合酶；诱生性一氧化氮合酶；诱生型一氧化氮合成酶；一氧化氮合成酶
Inflammatory biomarkers of stroke; Inflammatory biomarker of stroke; Inflammation indicators; Inflammatory indicators; Inflammatory indicator; Inflammation indicator; Inflammatory markers; Inflammation markers; Inflammation marker	脑卒中的炎症标志物

续　表

英文术语	中文术语
Inflammatory disorder; inflammatory disorders; Infectious disease; Infective disorder; Infectious disease (disorder); Infection; Inflammatory disease; Inflammatory disorder (disorder)	炎性疾病；感染；感染性疾病；感染病；炎症性疾病
Inflammatory mediators of secondary brain damage; Inflammatory mediators	继发性脑损伤的炎症介质；炎症介质
Inflammatory response; inflammation; Inflammatory responces; Inflammatory mechanism; Inflammatory reaction; Inflammatory pathway; Neuroinflammation; Inflammation	炎症；炎性反应
inflammatory response pathway; CLR signaling pathway	炎症反应途径
Inherited hypercoagulable condition; Hereditary hypercoagulable state	遗传性高凝状态
inosine; Increase of inosine	肌苷；次黄苷；肌甙；次黄嘌呤核苷；肌苷增加
Inpatient Rehabilitation Facilities; IRFs; Hospital rehabilitation institutions	住院康复机构；住院复健机构
Insomnia; Sleeplessness; insomnia; Sleep Initiation and Maintenance Disorders; agrypnia; Insomnia (disorder)	失眠；失眠症；入睡和保持睡眠障碍；入睡和睡眠障碍；失眠障碍
Instrumental Activities of Daily Living; intellect activities of daily living; instrumental activities of daily living	工具性日常生活活动；日常生活的工具性活动
Insulin resistance; Insulin Sensitivity; Insulin resistance in diabetes; Drug resistance to insulin; Drug resistance to insulin (disorder); Insulin resistance in diabetes (disorder)	胰岛素抵抗；胰岛素耐药；胰岛素抗药性
integrin subunit alpha 1; ITGA1	整合素 α1 亚基
Intention tremor; intentional tremor	意向性震颤；意向震颤
Inter-α-trypsin inhibitor heavy chain H3	胰蛋白酶抑制剂重链 H3
Intercellular Adhesion Molecule 1; soluble vascular cellular adhesion molecule 1; Intercellular Adhesion Molecule-1; Cluster of Differentiation 54; sVCAM-1; ICAM-1; CD-54	细胞间黏附分子 1
Interenal carotid artery atherosclerosis; Intercervical atherosclerosis; Intercervical arteriosclerosis; Intercervical atherosclerotic; Intercervical atheromatous; Intercervical artery atherosclerosis; Intercervical aortic atherosclerosis; Intercervical accelerated atherosclerosis; Intercervical coronary atherosclerosis	颈内动脉粥样硬化；颈间动脉粥样硬化；颈内动脉粥样硬化斑块

续　表

英文术语	中文术语
Interleukin 1; IL 1; IL-1; IL1; interleukin-1	白细胞介素 -1
Interleukin 1 beta; IL-1b; IL-1β; IL1β; IL1b	白细胞介素 1 β
Interleukin 10; interleukin-10; IL-10; IL10	白细胞介素 -10
Interleukin 18; IL 18; IL-18	白细胞介素 -18
Interleukin 23; IL12B; IL-23; IL23	白细胞介素 -23
Interleukin 6; IL 6; IL-6	白细胞介素 -6；α 白介素 6；白介素 -6
Internal carotid artery; Internal carotid arteries; ICAs; ICA; arteria carotis interna; internal carotid artery	颈内动脉
Internal carotid artery dissection; internal carotid artery dissection; Dissection of internal carotid artery; Internal carotid artery dissection (disorder); Dissection of internal carotid artery (disorder); ICAD	颈内动脉夹层
Internal carotid artery infarction syndrome; syndromes of internal carotid artery infarction; syndrome of internal carotid artery infarction; Internal carotid artery infarction syndromes; Internal carotid artery infarction symptom	颈内动脉梗死综合征
international classification of functioning, disability and health; World Health Organizaion's ICF; ICF	国际功能、残疾和健康分类
International normalized ratio; INR; international standardized ratio; international normal ratio	国际标准比值；国际化标准比值；国际标准化率；国际规格化比值
Interval; spacing; pause	间隔；间期；区间
intonation training; Tone training; utterance training	语调训练；音准训练
Intra-arterial thrombolysis; Intravascular thrombolysis; IA thrombolysis	血管内溶栓；动脉内取栓；动脉内溶栓术
Intraarterial Recombinant Tissue Plasminogen Activator; IA r-tPA; IA tPA	动脉内组织纤溶酶原激活剂；动脉内重组组织纤溶酶原激活剂
Intracranial sinus thrombosis; Cranial sinus thrombosis; Sinus Thrombosis	颅内窦血栓形成；颅窦血栓形成；静脉窦血栓形成
Intracranial thrombosis; cranial venous sinus thrombosis; intracranial thrombotic; intracranial venous sinus thrombosis; intracranial sinus thrombosis; cerebral thrombosis	颅内血栓形成；颅内血栓；颅内动脉闭塞；脑血栓

续　表

英文术语	中文术语
Intravenous Recombinant Tissue Plasminogen Activator; Intravenous tissue-type plasminogen activator; IV r-tPA; IV tPA	静脉重组组织纤溶酶原激活剂
Intravenous thrombolysis; IV thrombolysis	静脉溶栓；静脉溶栓治疗；静脉内溶栓；经静脉溶栓
intrinsic apoptotic pathway	内源性凋亡通路；内源性凋亡途径；内在凋亡途径；外源性信号途径
Intrinsic pathway	内源性途径；内在途径；内在通路；内途径；内在路径；内源途径；内凋亡途径；内源性通路
Ion gradient loss; ion-exchange gradient loss; ions gradient loss; ion solution gradient loss	离子梯度损失
Ipsilateral conjugate gaze palsy; Conjugated ipsilateral gaze paralysis	同侧共轭注视麻痹；眼侧共轭注视麻痹；同侧共轭注视轻瘫
Ipsilateral facial hemiplegia	同侧面部偏瘫
Ipsilateral facial hypesthesia; Ipsilateral facial hypalgesia	同侧面部感觉减退
Ipsilateral facial pain	同侧面部疼痛；患侧面部疼痛；患侧面部痛；同侧面部痛
Ipsilateral facial paralysis; Ipsilateral facial paresis	同侧面瘫；同侧性面瘫
Ipsilateral gait ataxia; Ipsilateral Ataxia of gait; Ipsilateral ataxic gait	同侧步态共济失调；单侧步态共济失调；一侧步态共济失调
Ipsilateral hearing loss; Ipsilateral deafness	同侧听力丧失；同侧听力损失
Ipsilateral lateropulsion	同侧步
Ipsilateral limb ataxia; ipsilateral limb defective coordination; ipsilateral limb incoordination	同侧肢体共济失调；一侧肢体共济失调；单侧肢体共济失调
Ipsilateral loss of taste; Loss of ipsilateral taste	同侧味觉丧失；同侧味觉障碍；同侧味觉缺陷；同侧味丧失
Ipsilateral nystagmus	同侧眼球震颤
Ipsilateral oculomotor paresis; ipsilateral oculomotor nerve paralysis; ipsilateral ocular nerve palsy; ipsilateral oculomotor palsy	同侧动眼神经麻痹；眼外侧动眼神经麻痹；一侧动眼神经麻痹
Ipsilateral third cranial nerve palsy; Ipsilateral oculomotor nerve palsy	同侧第三颅神经麻痹；患侧第三颅神经麻痹

续　表

英文术语	中文术语
Ipsilateral tongue paralysis; Ipsilateral hemiparalysis of tongue; Ipsilateral tongue paresis	同侧舌肌麻痹；舌侧麻痹
IQ motif containing GTPase activation protein 1; IQ motif-containing GTPase activation protein 1; IQGAP1	含有GTPase激活蛋白1的IQ基序
Ischemic modified albumin; Ischaemic modified albumin; IMA	缺血修饰白蛋白
Isolated ataxia	孤立性共济失调；孤立性运动失调
Isolated dysarthria	孤立性构音障碍；孤立性构音不良；孤立性构音困难
Isolated monoparesis; Isolated single limb paralysis	孤立单肢轻瘫；孤立单肢不全麻痹
Isometric tremor; Isoaxial tremor	等轴性震颤；等长收缩性震颤；等轴震颤；等距离震颤
Jak-Stat signaling pathway	酪氨酸蛋白激酶/信号转导子和转录激活子信号通路；JAK-STAT通路信号
Janus kinase 2; JAK2	Janus激酶2
Japan stroke scale; JSS	日本卒中评定表
joint activity training; range of motion training of whole joint; joint mobility training	关节活动度训练；联合活动训练
Juice; consumption of juice	果汁(或菜汁)饮料；果汁；果汁饮料
Katz index	Katz指数
Kawasaki syndrome; Acute febrile mucocutaneous lymph node syndrome; Kawasakis mucocutaneous lymph node syndrome; Kawasaki's disease; MCLS; MLNS; Mucocutaneous lymph node syndrome; Kawasaki's syndrome; Acute febrile mucocutaneous lymph node syndrome (disorder); Kawasaki disease	川崎综合征；急性发热性皮肤黏膜淋巴结综合征；川崎病；川崎综合征；粘膜皮肤淋巴结综合征；皮肤黏膜淋巴结综合征；小儿皮肤黏膜淋巴结综合征；皮肤-黏膜-淋巴结综合征；黏膜皮肤淋巴结综合征；急性发热性黏膜皮肤淋巴结综合征；皮肤黏膜淋巴结综合症；皮肤粘膜淋巴结综合征；川崎病(粘膜皮肤淋巴结综合征)；伴指(趾)特异性脱屑急性发热性皮肤黏膜淋巴结综合征；急性发热性皮肤粘膜淋巴结综合征(MCLS)；川崎氏病；Kawasaki病〔川崎病〕；急性发热性皮肤粘膜淋巴结综合征（MCLS）；Kawasaki综合征；小儿川崎病

续　表

英文术语	中文术语
Kinetic tremor	运动性震颤
Lack of spontaneity; verbal adynamia	自发性行为缺乏；自发性行为缺失
Lacunar infarction (disorder); Small vessel disorder; Penetrating artery disease; Small vessel disease; Lacunar infarction; Lacunar stroke; lacunar infarction; lacunar cerebral infarction; LACI - Lacunar infarction; LI - Lacunar infarction	腔隙性脑梗死；腔隙梗塞；腔隙性脑梗塞；腔隙性梗塞；腔隙性中风
Lacunar stroke syndrome; syndromes of lacunar stroke; syndrome of lacunar stroke; Lacunar stroke syndromes; LACS	腔隙性脑梗死症状
Large central visual field defect; Central large visual field defectCentral large visual field defects	中心视野缺损较大；大中心视野缺损；中央大视野缺损
Large vessel atherosclerosis; atherosclerosis; Atherosclerosis of artery; Atheroma of artery; Atheroma of artery (disorder); Large vessel atherosclerotic plaque; Large artery atherosclerosis; Atherosclerosis; LAA; Atherosclerosis artery; Atherosclerosis of artery (disorder)	大动脉粥样硬化；动脉粥样硬化；动脉粥样斑块；动脉粥样硬化斑块形成；大动脉粥样硬化斑块；动脉粥样硬化性动脉；粥样硬化性动脉
Large vessel disorder; great vessels diseases; macrovascular diseases; macrovascular disease; Large vessel disease	大血管疾病
Laryngeal dystonia; laryngeal dystonia; Laryngeal dystonia (disorder)	喉部肌张力障碍；喉肌张力障碍；咽肌张力障碍
Lauric acid; dodecanoic acid	月桂酸；十二烷酸；壳聚糖-月桂酸偶联物；椰油酸；十二酸
legumes; beans; bean; bean pods; leguminosae	豆类；豆科植物；杂豆；豆科作物；豆
Leisure and recreation activities; Recreational and Leisure Activity; Entertainment and leisure activities; recreation and leisure activities; recreational and leisure activities	休闲娱乐活动
Leukoaraiosis; Leuko-araiosis (finding); Periventricular white matter disease; Leuko-araiosis	脑白质病变；脑室周围白质病；脑白质缺血(放射影象征)
leuleuenkephalin; leucine; leucine-rich；leukin；l-leucine；L-leucine; leonine acid; Increase of leuleuenkephalin	亮氨酸；亮氨酸增加
Lewy bodies	Lewy 小体；路易体；Lewy 体
Licostinel; ACEA 1021	利可替奈
life self-care; self-care; life-independent; living self-care; self-help	生活自理

英文术语	中文术语
Life style modification; lifestyle change; living style change; behavior change	生活方式改变；生活方式的修改；生活方式改进
Limb apraxia; Limb kinetic apraxia	肢体失用；肢体失用症；肢体失语
Limb ataxia	肢体共济失调
Limb dysmetria; Poor limb distance discrimination	肢体辨距不良；肢体辨距障碍；肢距离辨别障碍
Limb dystonia	肢体肌张力障碍
Limb shaking TIA; limb shaking transient ischemic attack	肢体抖动性短暂性脑缺血发作；肢体抖动短暂性脑缺血发作
Limb tremor; limbs tremor	肢体震颤；四肢震颤
Line Bisection test; Tests of visual inattention	线段等分试验；线等分试验
lipid metabolic pathway; lipid metabolism	脂质代谢途径；脂代谢途径；脂类代谢途径
Lipid metabolism; fat metabolism; lipometabolism; metabolism, lipid; lipid metabolic; lipid; fatty metabolism; lipid metabolize	脂质代谢；脂代谢；脂肪代谢；脂类代谢；血脂代谢；糖脂代谢；
Lipid oxidation; fatty acid oxidation	脂质氧化；脂肪酸氧化；脂肪氧化；油脂氧化；脂氧化
Lipid peroxidation; lipid peroxides; lipid oxidation; lipid peroxidate; membrane lipid peroxidation; lipids peroxidation; anti-lipid peroxidation	脂质过氧化；脂过氧化；脂质过氧化作用；脂过氧化作用；脂质过氧化反应；脂质过氧化物；过氧化脂质；膜质过氧化
lipidomics biomarkers of stroke	脑卒中的脂质组学生物标志物
Lipohyalinosis; lipoproteinemia; Fibrinoid necrosis	脂质玻璃样变；脂蛋白血症；纤维蛋白样坏死
lipopolysaccharide binding protein; BPIFD2; LBP	脂多糖结合蛋白
Lipoprotein a; Lipoprotein(a); Lp(a)	脂蛋白(a)；脂蛋白类；血清脂蛋白；血清(a)
Lipoprotein associated phospholipase A2; Platelet-activating factor acetylhydrolase; Lipoprotein-associated phospholipase A2; LDL-associated phospholipase A2; PAF acetylhydrolase; LDL-PLA2; Lp-PLA2; PLA2G7	脂蛋白相关磷酯酶A2
Lipoprotein oxidation	脂蛋白氧化修饰；脂蛋白氧化；ldl氧化

英文术语	中文术语
Local percutaneous electrical stimulation; Local transcutaneous electrical nerve stimulation; Local transcutaneous electrical acustimulation; Local transcutaneous electric stimulation; Local transcutaneous electric nerve stimulation; Local transcutaneous electrical stimulation therapy; Local transcutaneous electroacupuncture	局部经皮电刺激
Locked in syndrome; Lockedin syndrome; locked-in syndrome; LiS; LIS; Locked in syndrome (disorder)	闭锁综合征；闭锁综合症；闭锁症候群；闭锁综合症（Locked-In）
Logorrhea; Logorrhoea; Logorrhea (finding); Press of speech	多语症；多言癖
Long-term Acute Care Hospitals; Long term acute nursing hospital; Long term acute care hospital	长期急症护理医院；长期急性护理医院
Loss of corneal reflex; Decreased corneal reflex; Reduced corneal reflex; Decreased blink reflex	角膜反射减少
Loss of pain; Decreased pain sensation; Impaired pain sensation	痛觉消失；痛觉障碍
Loss of temperature; Abnormality of temperature sensation; Impaired temperature sensation; Loss of temperature sensation	温度觉障碍；温觉障碍
Lovastatin	洛伐他汀
Low birth weight; History of low birth weight; Low birth weight infant; LBW - Low birth weight infant; Low birth weight infant (disorder)	低体重儿；低出生体重儿；低出生体重；低出生体重新生儿；低出生体重婴儿；低体重新生儿；低体重婴儿；新生儿低体重；婴儿低出生体重
low density lipoprotein cholesterol; LDL-C	低密度脂蛋白胆固醇；低密度胆固醇；低密度脂蛋白
Low glycaemic index diet intake; Glycemic index of the diet; Low glycaemic index food; Glycemic index	低血糖指数饮食摄入
Low hemoglobin level; Low hemoglobin levels	血红蛋白下降；血红蛋白水平低；血红蛋白含量低
Low molecular weight heparins; LMWH; low molecular weight heparin; low molecular weight heparins; low molecular weight heparin calcium; low molecule weight heparin; low molecular heparin sodium; low-molecular mass; lower molecule heparin	低分子肝素；低分子量肝素
low triglyceride level; low serum triglyceride level; low serum triglyceride	低甘油三酯水平

续　表

英文术语	中文术语
Low-density lipoprotein; Low density lipoprotein; Bad cholesterol; LDL	低密度脂蛋白；低密度胆固醇；低密度酯蛋白胆固醇
Low-to-normal blood pressure; Low to normal blood pressure	血压低至正常；低至正常血压
Lower Extremity Strengthening; Lower limb reinforcement training; lower extremity reinforcement training; membrum inferius reinforcement training; lower limb reinforcement training; lower limbs reinforcement training; limb reinforcement training; leg reinforcement training; Lower limb enhancement training; lower extremity enhancement training; membrum inferius enhancement training; lower limb enhancement training; lower limbs enhancement training; limb enhancement training; leg enhancement training	下肢增强训练；下肢强化
Lower extremity weakness; Leg weakness; Muscle weakness in lower limbs; Lower limb weakness	下肢无力；瘫脚病；腿病
lower limb strength; lower extremity muscle strength; muscle strength of lower limbs; muscle strength of lower extremities; extremity muscle strength; muscular strength of lower limbs; lower extremity muscle; lower limb muscle strength	下肢肌力；下肢肌肉力量
Lubeluzole; R-91154	芦贝鲁唑
lymphocyte antigen 96; LY96	淋巴细胞抗原96
Macronutrient intake; Macronutrients; Macronutrient	宏量营养素摄入
Macrophage; Macrophages; macrophage; macrophages; macrophage cell; macrophage cells; macrophagocyte; alveolar macrophage; phagocyte; microphage; Macrophage activation	巨噬细胞；巨噬细胞活化
Magnesium; Mg; magnesium	镁
Magnesium deficiency; magnesium deficiency; Hypomagnesaemia; hypomagnesemia; hypomagnesaemia; Hypomagnesiuria; Hypomagnesemia; Hypomagnesemia (disorder); Magnesium deficiency (disorder)	低镁血症；镁缺乏；低血镁症；镁缺乏症；镁代谢失常综合症
Magnetic resonance angiography; MR angiography; MRA	磁共振血管成像
Magnetic resonance imaging; MRI; magnetic resonance image; magnetic resonance; magnetic resonance spectroscopy; magnetic resonance angiography	磁共振成像；磁共振；核磁共振成像；核磁共振；磁共振影像

英文术语	中文术语
malnutrition; Poor nutritional status; undernourishment; nutritional inadequacy; faulty nutrition; nutrition; nutrition, defective; inadequate nutrition; underfeeding	营养不良；营养不足
Malondialdehyde; MDA	丙二醛（MDA）
Managing money; financial management; finance; financial; wealth management; money managment; finance management; financial planning; personal finance	理财；管理钱财
Mannitol	甘露醇；己六醇；甘露糖醇
manual function score; MFS	偏瘫手功能评分；手动功能评分
Marfan syndrome; Marfan's syndrome; Marfan's disease; Marfan's syndrome (disorder)	马凡综合征；马方综合征；Marfan综合征
Margarine intake; margarine	人造奶油摄入量；人造黄油摄入量；人造黄油摄入
Marie Foix syndrome; Lateral pontine syndrome	脑桥外侧综合征；玛丽海绵窦综合征
massage; Chinese traditional manipulation	按摩；推拿；按摩术
Mast cell expressed membrane protein 1; chromosome 19 open reading frame 59; C19ORF59; MCEMP1	肥大细胞表达膜蛋白1
Mathew stroke scale	马修卒中量表；Mathew中风量表
Matrix metalloproteinase 1; Matrix metalloproteinase-1; MMP 1; MMP-1; MMP1	基质金属蛋白酶1；金属基质蛋白酶1；金属蛋白酶1；金属蛋白酶组织抑制因子1；血清基质金属蛋白酶1
Matrix metalloproteinase 13; Matrix metalloproteinase-13; MMP-13; MMP 13; MMP13	基质金属蛋白酶13(MMP-13)；基质金属蛋白酶13；金属基质蛋白酶13；金属蛋白酶13；基质金属蛋白13；血清基质金属蛋白酶13
Matrix metalloproteinase 2; Matrix metalloproteinase-2; MMP-2; MMP 2; MMP2	基质金属蛋白酶2；金属基质蛋白酶2；金属蛋白酶2；血清基质金属蛋白酶2；基质金属蛋白激酶2
Matrix metalloproteinase 3; Matrix metalloproteinase-3; MMP 3; MMP-3; MMP3	基质金属蛋白酶3；金属基质蛋白酶3；金属蛋白酶3；基质金属蛋白3；血清基质金属蛋白酶3

续　表

英文术语	中文术语
Matrix metalloproteinase 9; Matrix metalloproteinase-9; MMP 9; MMP-9; MMP9	基质金属蛋白酶9；金属基质蛋白酶9；金属蛋白酶9；基质金属蛋白9；血清基质金属蛋白酶9
Matrix metalloproteinases; MMPs; MMP	基质金属蛋白酶；金属基质蛋白酶；金属蛋白酶；金属蛋白酶类；基质金属蛋白；血清基质金属蛋白酶
Measurement of body mass index; measurement of BMI; BMI measurements; BMI measurement	体重指数测量；体质指数测量；BMI测量
Measures of comorbidity; Comorbidity Index	共病措施；共病指数
Mechanical Clot Disruption; Mechanical clot retrieval	机械性血栓破裂
Mechanical Clot Extraction	机械性血栓提取；机械凝块提取
Mechanical thrombectomy	机械取栓；机械血栓清除；机械溶栓；机械取栓术；机械碎栓；机械血栓切除术
Mechanisms of atherosclerotic cerebrovascular disease; stroke pathogenesis; Etiology of atherosclerotic cerebrovascular disease	动脉粥样硬化性脑血管病的发病机制；动脉粥样硬化性脑血管病的病因；动脉粥样硬化性脑血管病病因；动脉粥样硬化性脑血管病发病机制
Medial medullary infarction symptom; Infarction of medial medulla; Dejerine syndrome; MMI	延髓内侧综合征
medical examination	体格检查；内科检查；医学检查；医疗检查
Medical Research Council	MRC法
Medications for Motor Recovery; Exercise recovery drug therapy; motion recovery drug therapy; sports recovery drug therapy; motor recovery drug therapy; Exercise recovery drug treatment; motion recovery drug treatment; sports recovery drug treatment; motor recovery drug treatment; Exercise recovery medication; motion recovery medication; sports recovery medication; motor recovery medication; Exercise recovery pharmacotherapy; motion recovery pharmacotherapy; sports recovery pharmacotherapy; motor recovery pharmacotherapy	运动恢复药物治疗；运动恢复药物疗法
Mediterranean diet	地中海饮食；地中海式饮食

英文术语	中文术语
melodic intonation therapy; MIT	旋律语调疗法；MIT法；旋律语调法；旋律发音治疗；音乐音调治疗法；旋律音调治疗；旋律语调治疗；旋律音调疗法
Memory; memory abilities; remembrance; memorization; memorized; memories; remember; recollection; memory	记忆；记忆力
Memory loss; Loss of memory	记忆丧失；记忆缺失；失忆
mendelsohn method; Mendelsohn maneuver	门德尔松手法；门德尔松吞咽法
Metabolic disease; metabolic disorder; MD - Metabolic disorders; Metabolic disease (disorder); Metabolic disorders; Metabolic diseases; Metabolic disorder	代谢性疾病；代谢紊乱；代谢失调；代谢病；代谢性病症；代谢疾病
Metabolic syndrome; Metabolic syndrome X; Dysmetabolic syndrome X; Reaven's syndrome; Metabolic syndrome X (disorder)	代谢综合征；X综合征；代谢性综合症；代谢综合症；代谢综合征X；胰岛素抵抗综合征；代谢紊乱综合征；X代谢综合征
Metamorphopsia; metamorphopsia; Distortion of visual image; Distortion of visual image (disorder)	视物变形；视物变形症；视觉变形
Metformin; Diaformin Metformin; diaformin; dimethylbiguanide	二甲双胍；盐酸二甲双胍；降糖片
Microalbuminuria; microalbuminuria; moderately increased albuminuria; Moderately increased albuminuria; Microalbuminuria (finding)	微量白蛋白尿；微量蛋白尿；微白蛋白尿
Microatheromas; microaneurysm; microaneurysms	微动脉瘤；微小动脉瘤；小动脉瘤；微血管瘤；微脉瘤；微型动脉瘤
Microcirculatory dysfunction; microcirculation disturbance; microcirculatory disturbance; microcirculation disorder; microcirculation dysfunction; microcirculatory disorder; obstacle of microcirculation; microvascular dysfunction	微循环障碍
Microembolism; microthrombosis; microcirculation	微栓塞；微栓子；微小脑梗死灶
Microglia cell; Microgliocyte; Gitter cell	小神经胶质细胞；格子细胞
Microscopic polyangitis; microscopic polyangiitis	显微镜下多血管炎；显微镜下型多血管炎
Microvascular dysfunction; microvessel dysfunction; coronary microvascular dysfunction	微血管功能障碍；微循环障碍；微血管病变；微血管损伤；微血管障碍

续　表

英文术语	中文术语
Midbrain; midbrain	中脑
Midbrain infarction symptom; Mesencephalic stroke	中脑梗死综合征；中脑梗死症状；中脑卒中
Middle cereberal artery infarction syndrome; syndromes of middle cereberal artery infarction; syndrome of middle cereberal artery infarction; Middle cereberal artery infarction syndromes; Middle cereberal artery infarction symptom; MCA infarction symptom; Sylvian artery	大脑中动脉梗死综合征
Middle cerebral artery; middle cerebral artery; Middle cerebral arteries; MCAs; MCA	大脑中动脉
Middle cerebral artery atherosclerosis; Middle cerebral atherosclerotic plaque; middle artery atherosclerosis; middle cerebral arterial atherosclerosis; middle cerebral atherosclerosis; cerebral middle artery atherosclerosis; middle celebral artery atherosclerosis; cerebrum median artery atherosclerosis	大脑中动脉粥样硬化；大脑中动脉粥样硬化斑块
Migraine; migraine; megrim; Sick headache; Sick headache (disorder); Migraine (disorder)	偏头痛；偏头疼
Migraine with aura; Classical migraine; Migraine with aura (disorder)	先兆偏头痛；有先兆偏头痛；典型偏头痛；有典型先兆的偏头痛(经典型偏头痛)；经典型偏头痛；有先兆的偏头痛；先兆型偏头痛
Migraine without aura; Migraine without aura (disorder)	无先兆偏头痛；偏头痛不伴先兆；普通型偏头痛；无先兆的偏头痛；无先兆型偏头痛；无先兆性偏头痛；没有先兆的偏头痛
Migrainous infarction; Migrainous stroke; Migraine cerebral infarction	偏头痛性脑梗死；偏头痛性中风；偏头痛型梗塞
Mild contralateral hemiparesis	轻度对侧偏瘫
Millard Gubler syndrome; Ventral pontine syndrome	脑桥腹外侧综合征；静脉桥综合征
mimics	模型
Mini-Mental State Examination; mini mental status examination; MMSE	简易精神状态检查量表；简明智能状态检查量表
Mini-Mental Status Exam	微型精神状态检查；微小精神状态检查

续 表

英文术语	中文术语
Minocycline; minocycline hydrochloride; Klinomycin; Minocin; Minocyn; Vectrin Minocycline	米诺环素；美满霉素；盐酸米诺环素
Miosis; Constricted pupil; Miotic pupil; miosis; Pupil constriction; Constricted pupil (finding)	瞳孔缩小；瞳孔收缩
Misjudgment; erroneous decision; erroneous judgement; misidentification; misjudgement; misjudge; faulty judgement; erroneous judgment	判决失当；判断错误；错案；误判
Mitochondrial cytopathy; Mitochondrial disease; Mitochondrial myopathy; Mitochondrial cytopathy (disorder)	线粒体细胞病；线粒体病；线粒体疾病
Mitochondrial damage; Mitochondrial DNA disease; mtDNA mutation; mtDNA disease	线粒体损伤；线粒体DNA病；线粒体DNAT突变
Mitochondrial encephalopathy; Mitochondrial myopathy, encephalopathy lactic acidosis and stroke like episodes; Mitochondrial myopathy, encephalopathy lactic acidosis and stroke-like episodes; mitochondrial encephalomyopathy; MELAS; mitochondrial encephalopathy; Mitochondrial encephalomyopathy; Mitochondrial myoencephalopathy; Mitochondrial encephalomyopathy (disorder)	线粒体脑病；线粒体脑肌病；线粒体性脑肌病
Mitochondrial toxicity; mitochondria toxicity	线粒体毒性
Mitogen activated protein kinase; MAPK	丝裂原激活蛋白激酶；钙调蛋白依赖性蛋白激酶；促丝裂原蛋白活化激酶；丝裂原蛋白激酶；p38丝裂原活化蛋白激酶；丝裂原活化蛋白激酶；丝裂原活化蛋白激酶链
Mitogen-Activated Protein Kinase Signaling Pathway; MAPK signaling pathway	丝裂原活化蛋白激酶信号通路
Modifiable risk factors; Modifiable risk factor; Variable risk factors; Variable risk factor	可改变的风险因素；可控制的危险因素；可改变的危险因素；可改变的影响因素；可改变的高危因素；可改变的风险因子
Modification of a primary serum lipid biomarker; Modification of a major lipid biomarker	一种主要血脂生物标志物的修饰；原发性血脂生物标志物的修饰
modified Ashworth scale	改良Ashworth量表；改良的Ashworth分级

续　表

英文术语	中文术语
Modified Rankin Scale; Rankin Scale; mRS	改良 Rankin 量表
Molecular biomarkers of stroke; Cerebrospinal fluid biomarkers of stroke; Cellular biomarkers of stroke; Molecular biomarker of stroke; Cellular biomarker of stroke; Plasma biomarkers of stroke; Serum biomarkers of stroke; Blood biomarkers of stroke; Serum biomarker of stroke; Blood biomarker of stroke	脑卒中的分子标志物
Molecular mediators; Molecular medium	分子介质；分子介体
monocarboxylic acid transporter	单羧酸转运体
Monoclonal antibodies; monoclonal antibodies; murine intercellular adhesion molecule-1 antibody; Anti-ICAM-1 monoclonal antibody R6.5; murine ICAM-1 antibody	单克隆抗体类
Monocular horizontal nystagmus; ocellus horizontal nystagmus	单眼水平性眼球震颤；单侧水平性眼球震颤
Monocyte; mononuclear cell; monocytes; monocytic; human monocytes; human monocyte; mononuclear cells; Mon monocyte; monocyte	单核细胞
Monocyte chemoattractant protein 1; Recombinant Monocyte Chemoattractant Protein-1; Monocyte chemoattractant protein-1; Chemokine CCL2; MCP1	单核细胞趋化因子-1；趋化因子 CCL2；重组单核细胞趋化蛋白-1
Monounsaturated fatty acid; MUFA	单不饱和脂肪酸
Morning myoclonic jerks	早晨肌阵挛样抽动
Motor Assessment Scale	运动评估量表；卒中患者运动功能评估量表；运动评分法；运动功能评定量表
motor dysfunction; Motor deficit; motor disturbance; disturbance of motion; motor disorders; motor disorder; movement disorders; motility disorders	运动障碍；运动缺陷；肢体运动障碍；运动功能障碍
Motor Evaluation Scale for Upper Extremity in Stroke Patients; MESUPES-hand test; MESUPES-arm test; MESUPES	脑卒中患者上肢运动评价量表
motor function; movement function; motion function; motility function; activity function; movement ability; motor ability	运动功能；运动机能；运动能力；肢体功能；肢体运动功能
Motor hemineglect; Half-side motion neglect; Motion half side neglect	运动性忽略症；运动半侧忽略；运动偏身忽略；半侧运动忽略

续　表

英文术语	中文术语
motor imagery; motor imaginary therapy; active imagery therapy; exercise imagination therapy; mental practice; motion imaginary therapy; motor imagining therapy; motion imagination therapy; motor imagination therapy	运动想象疗法；运动想象；运动想像；运动表象
motor relearning program; sports relearning technology; motor relearning programme; MRP	运动再学习法；运动再学习方案；运动再学习疗法；运动再学习方法；运动再学习技术
Motor-Free Visual Perception Test; MVPT	无运动视觉感知测试
motricity index; MI	运动力指数；MI评测法
Movement; migration; translocation; shift; trans; shifting	移动；变动；转变；转移
Moyamoya disease; Familial moyamoya disease; Moyamoya syndrome; MMD; moyamoya disease; Carotid artery insufficiency syndrome; Progressive intracranial arterial occlusion; Taveras' syndrome; Moyamoya disease (disorder)	烟雾病；脑底异常血管网病；烟雾综合征；云雾病；颅底异常血管网病；moyamoya病；脑底异常血管网；云雾病(脑底异常血管网病)
mTOR signaling pathway	mTOR信号通路；mTOR通路；mTOR信号途径；PI3K/Akt/mTOR信号通路；哺乳动物雷帕霉素靶蛋白信号通路；mTOR信号传导通路
Multimodal facial hypaethesia; Multimodal facial sensory disturbance; Multimodal facial sensation disorders; Multimodal facial sensation disorder; Multimodal facial sensation disturbance	多模式面部感觉减退；多模式面部感觉障碍；多模式面部感觉缺失；多模式面部感觉缺陷
Multimodal reperfusion therapy; MMRT	多模式再灌注治疗；多模态再灌注治疗；多模态再灌注疗法
Multiphase CTA; Multi-phase CTA; mCTA	多相CTA
Multiple sclerosis; Disseminated sclerosis; MS; Multiple Sclerosis; multiple sclerosis; Generalised multiple sclerosis; Generalized multiple sclerosis; DS - Disseminated sclerosis; MS - Multiple sclerosis; Multiple sclerosis (disorder)	多发性硬化；多发性硬化症；多发性脑脊髓硬化症；脑脊髓多发性硬化；脑脊髓多发性硬化症
muscle tone; muscular tone; muscle tonus; muscle tensio; muscular tension; Muscle tension	肌张力；肌紧张；肌张力的；肌肉紧张；肌紧张度；肌拉力
Myelin basic protein; MBP	髓鞘碱性蛋白；甘露糖结合蛋白
Myocardial infarction	心肌梗死
Myoclonic spasms	肌阵挛性抽搐

续　表

英文术语	中文术语
Myoclonus; myoclonus; Myoclonia; Myoclonus (finding)	肌阵挛
Myristic acid; Tetradecanoic Acid	肉豆蔻酸；十四酸；豆蔻酸；十四烷酸
N acetylaspartate; N-acetyl-L-aspartate; N-acetylaspartate; NAA	N乙酰天冬氨酸
N acetylneuraminate pyruvate lyase; CHROMOSOME 1 OPEN READING FRAME 13; N-acetylneuraminate pyruvate lyase; C1ORF13	N乙酰神经氨酸丙酮酸裂解酶
N formyl peptide receptor; N-formyl peptide receptor	N甲酰肽受体
N glycan; N-glycan	N聚糖；糖苷；多糖
N methyl D aspartate receptor antagonists; N-methyl-D-aspartate receptor antagonists; Anti-NMDA receptor; Anti NMDA receptor; NMDA receptors; NMDA receptor; NMDAR; NR2; NR1	N甲基D天冬氨酸受体拮抗剂；N-甲基-D-天冬氨酸受体拮抗剂
N terminal proBNP; N-terminal pro-brain natriuretic peptide; N-terminal pro-BNP; N-BNP peptide; NBNP peptide; NT-proBNP	N末端脑钠肽前体
Nalmefene; Cervene	纳美芬；钠美芬；盐酸纳美芬
narcolepsy; Episodic hypersomnia	发作性睡病；发作性嗜睡；发作性睡眠过多
Narcotic receptor antagonist; Anesthetic receptor antagonists	麻醉性受体拮抗剂
Nasal, dysarthic speech; Nasal, articulation disorder; Nasal, articulation impediment; Nasal, articulation disorders	鼻，构音障碍；鼻音、构音障碍言语
National Institutes of Health Stroke Scale; National Institutes of Health Stroke Scale Ontology; NIHSS score; NIHSS; NIH stroke scale	美国国立卫生研究院卒中量表；美国国立卫生研究院脑卒中评定表
Nausea; nausea; Retching; Retching (finding); Nauseated; Nauseous; Nausea (finding)	恶心
Necrosis; Tissue devitalisation; Cellular necrosis	坏死；细胞坏死；组织分化
necrosis pathway; Pathway of necrosis	坏死途径
Necrotizing vasculitis; necrotizing vasculitis; Necrotizing angitis; Necrotising vasculitis; Necrotizing vasculitis (disorder)	坏死性血管炎；坏死性血管炎症；坏死性血管病(非特异性)；坏死性血管病变
neglect; ignores; neglects; overlooked; overlooks; disregard of; neglected; ignore	忽视；疏忽；忽略
Nerve pathway; path; route; way; approach; paths	神经传导通路；路径；途径；传导途径

英文术语	中文术语
Neuroanatomy	神经解剖；脑解剖；人脑解剖
Neurochemical changes; Neurochemical alter; Neurochemical transform; Neurochemical turn	神经化学改变
Neurofibromatosis type 1; NF1; Clinical von Reclinghausen's disease; Von Recklinghausen disease; Neurofibromatosis, peripheral type; Neurofibromatosis 1; NF1 - Neurofibromatosis type 1; Neurofibromatosis, type 1; Neurofibromatosis, type 1 (disorder); Neurofibromatosis type 1 (disorder)	1型神经纤维瘤病；神经纤维瘤病，外周型；神经纤维瘤病1型；神经纤维瘤病；神经纤维瘤病1；Von Recklinghausen病；1型神经纤维瘤
Neurofilament light protein; NFL	神经丝轻蛋白
Neurogenic bladder; neurogenic bladder; Neuropathic bladder; Neurogenic bladder (finding)	神经源性膀胱；神经原性膀胱；神经源性膀胱功能障碍；神经源性膀胱尿道功能障碍
Neuroimaging; neurography; neuroimage; neural-imaging	神经影像学；神经影像；脑功能成像；神经成像；神经显像
Neuroimaging biomarkers of stroke; Stroke imaging markers; Stroke imaging marker; SIM	脑卒中的神经影像学生物标志物
Neurological tests; Neurophysiological monitoring; Neurophysiological test; Neurologic evaluation; Neurological test	神经测试；神经试验
Neurology Department; neurological department; neurological internal medicine; neurological; neural department of internal medicine	神经内科病房；神经内科；精神科
neurology physician; neurologists; neurologist; Neurologists	神经内科医师；神经病学医生；神经科医生
Neuromuscular dysphagia; Neuromuscular dysphagy; Neuromuscular dyskinesia; Neuromuscular acataposis; Neuromuscular deglutitio impedita	神经肌肉源性吞咽困难；神经肌肉吞咽障碍
neuromuscular electrical stimulation; neuromuscular electric stimulation; neuromuscular electric stimulation therapy; electrical nerve stimulation; nerve muscle electrical stimulation; neuromuscular stimulation	神经肌肉电刺激；吞咽神经肌肉电刺激；仿生物电刺激；神经肌肉电刺激疗法；肌肉神经电刺激
Neuronal biomarkers of stroke; Neuronal biomarker of stroke	脑卒中的神经元生物标志物
Neurone specific enolase; NSE	神经元特异性烯醇化酶

续　表

英文术语	中文术语
neuropeptide Y; Increase of neuropeptide Y	神经肽 Y；血浆神经肽 Y；神经肽 Y(NPY)；血清神经肽 Y；脑肠肽酪神经肽；神经肽 Y 增加
Neuroprotective therapy; Neuroprotective drugs therapy; Neuroprotective agents; Neuroprotective drug therapy	神经保护治疗；神经保护药物治疗
Neuroserpin; Neuroserpin Polymorphisms	神经源性丝氨酸蛋白酶抑制剂
neurotensin; Increase of neurotensin	神经降压素；神经降压肽；神经加压素；神经紧张素；神经降压素(NT)；神经降压素增加
Niacin; NA; Nicotinic acid; nicotinic acid	烟酸；尼克酸
NIHSS Instruction	NIHSS 说明
NIHSS Report	NIHSS 报告
Nimodipine	尼莫地平
Nitric oxide; nitrogen monoxide; level of nitric oxide; nitrogen oxide; nitrous oxide; nitric oxid; nitric oxygen; nitro oxide ; NO	一氧化氮
nitric oxide synthase 3; ECNOS; eNOS; NOS3	一氧化氮合酶 3
Nitric oxide synthesis; Nitric oxid production; NO production; NO synthesis; Production of nitric oxide	一氧化氮合成；一氧化氮生成
Nitrosative stress	氮化应激；亚硝基化应激；亚硝酸化应激；硝化应激
NMDA autoantibodies; N-methyl D-aspartate autoantibodies; NMDA receptor autoantibodies; NMDA receptor antagonist; NR2A/2B antibodies; NR2A/2B Abs	N-甲基 D-天冬氨酸自身抗体
No evidence of DVT	无 DVT 的证据
No history of heart disease	无心脏病史；没有心脏病史
No serious arrhythmia	无严重的心律失常
nonbacterial intracranial venous thrombosis; nonbacterial cerebral venous thrombosis; Aseptic venous thrombosis; Aseptic intracranial venous thrombosis	非化脓性颅内静脉窦血栓形成；无菌性颅内静脉栓塞
Noncontrast MRA	非对比 MRA；非对比磁共振血管造影检查

英文术语	中文术语
Nonmodifiable risk factors; Nonmodifiable risk factor	不可改变的风险因素；不可改变的影响因素；不可改变的高危因素；不可调整的影响因素；不可调整的高危因素；不可调整的风险因素
Nonprogressive cerebellar ataxia	非进行性小脑性共济失调
Nonspecifc markers of coagulation; Nonspecifc marker of coagulation	凝血相关非特异性标志物
Nonspecific markers of stroke; Nonspecific marker of stroke	脑卒中的非特异性标志物
Notch signaling pathway	Notch信号通路；Notch信号途径；Notch通路；Notch信号；Notch信号转导通路
Nottingham Sensory Assessment	诺丁汉感官评定；诺丁汉感官评价；Nottingham感官评定
Nuclear factor kappa B; hepatic nuclear factor-kB; NF-kappa B; NF-kB; NF kB	核转录因子-kB；肝细胞核因子-kB
nuclear factor kappa B signaling pathway; NF-kappaB signaling pathway; NF-kB signaling pathway	核因子κB信号通路
nuclear factor, erythroid 2 like 2 signaling pathway; Nrf2 signaling pathway	核因子红细胞2相关因子2信号通路；核因子，红系2样2信号通路；核因子红样2相关因子2信号通路
Nucleoside diphosphate kinase A; NDKA	核苷二磷酸激酶a亚基
Nucleosomes; Nucleosome	核小体；核粒；核蛋白体
Nursing; nursing sciences; nursing care; care; nurse; nurses; clinical nursing; caring; nursing measure	护理；护理学
Nursing Homes; skilled nursing facility; nursing hospital; nursing home	疗养院；疗养所；养老院；养老机构；护养院；护理之家；休养所；护理院
Nutritional counseling; individualized nutritional counseling	营养咨询；营养辅导
Nutritionists; nutritionist; dietician; dietitian	营养师；营养学家
Nuts; walnut; nut fruit	坚果；果仁；坚果仁；干果
Nystagmus; nystagmus; Uncontrolled eye movements; Nystagmus (disorder)	眼球震颤；眼震；眼震颤
Nystagmus-induced head nodding; Nodding caused by eye tremor	眼球震颤诱发的点头运动；眼球震颤引起的点头

续　表

英文术语	中文术语
Obesity; Adiposity; Adiposis; Obese (finding); Obesity (disorder); obesity; fatty; adiposity; Obese; Morbid obesity; Morbid obesity (disorder)	肥胖；脂肪过多；肥胖(症)；肥胖病；体脂肪率；肥胖症；病态肥胖症；病态性肥胖；病态肥胖
Obstructive sleep apnea; Obstructive sleep apneas; OSA; Obstructive sleep apnea syndrome; Obstructive sleep apnoea syndrome; OSA - Obstructive sleep apnea; OSA - Obstructive sleep apnoea; Obstructive sleep apnea syndrome (disorder); Obstructive sleep apnoea; obstructive sleep apnea	阻塞性睡眠呼吸暂停综合症；阻塞性睡眠呼吸暂停综合征；阻塞性睡眠呼吸暂停
Occipital brain region	枕叶脑区
Occipital neuralgia; occipital neuralgia; Cervico-occipital neuralgia; Cervico-occipital neuralgia (finding)	枕神经痛；颈枕神经痛；颈枕部神经痛；枕部神经痛
Occipitocervical headache; Occipital headache	枕颈性头痛；枕颈头痛；枕颈部头痛
Occupational therapy; occupation therapy; operating therapy; operation treatment; work treatment	职业疗法；作业疗法；职能治疗；工疗；职业治疗；作业治疗学；职业治疗法；作业治疗技术
Occupational Therapy Adult Perceptual Screening Test; OT-APST	职业治疗成人知觉筛查试验
Ocular dyssynergia	眼协同失调
Ocular tilt reaction; Ocular deviation reaction	眼倾斜反应；眼偏斜反应
Oculogyric crisis; oculogyric crisis; Oculogyric crisis (finding)	动眼危象；动眼神经危象；眼动危象；眼球旋动危象
Oculomotor apraxia; Ocular apraxia; Oculomotor apraxia (disorder)	眼球运动不能；动眼运动异常；眼运动不能；眼球运动障碍
Olive oil; olive oils; azeite; virgin olive oil; olive	橄榄油
OMICS biomarkers of stroke; OMICS biomarker of stroke	卒中的组学生物标志物
Ondine syndrome; Sleep-related respiratory failure (disorder); Ondine's curse; Sleep-related respiratory failure; Ondine's curse	Ondine综合征；睡眠相关性呼吸衰竭
Onset of symptom; Symptom Onset	开始出现症状
Ontario Society of Occupational Therapists Perceptual Evaluation; OSOT Perceptual Evaluation	安大略职业治疗师学会感性评估
Optic ataxia; visuomotor apraxia	视觉性共济失调
Optical fiber velopharyngeal endoscopy	光纤维腭咽喉内镜

英文术语	中文术语
Optokinetic nystagmus	视旋转性眼球震颤；视动性眼球震颤；视觉运动性眼震；视动性眼震
Oral contraceptive pill; Oral contraception; Pill - oral contraception; OC - Oral contraceptive; Oral contraception (finding); Oral contraceptives; Oral contraceptive; OCs; OCP	口服避孕药；服药避孕
Oral function evaluation; Oral functional estimate; Oral functions evaluation; Oral function valuation; Oral functional evaluation; Oral functional assessment; Oral functional appraisal; Oral evaluation	口腔功能评价；口面功能评价
Oral-pharyngeal dysphagia; Oropharyngeal dysphagia; Pharyngeal dysphagia; Transfer dysphagia; Oropharyngeal dysphagia (disorder)	口咽部吞咽困难；口咽吞咽困难；口咽部吞咽障碍；口咽吞咽障碍
organization; institutional; institution; agencies; institute; organ; apparatus; association; mechanism; machine; agency	机构；制度；制度环境
Orgogozo stroke scale	奥戈佐卒中量表；Orgogozo卒中量表
Orofacial dyskinesia; Orofacial dyskinesia (disorder)	口面运动障碍；口面部运动障碍；运动障碍(口面部)
Oromandibular dystonia	口下颌肌张力障碍
Oromotor apraxia; Dysphasia; Disorder of language (finding); dysphasia; Discourse disorder; Verbal dyspraxia; Disorder of language; DYSPHASIA; Language impairment; Dysphasia (finding); Verbal dyspraxia (disorder); Discourse disorder (disorder)	语言障碍；言语障碍症；言语障碍；语言困难；话语障碍
oropharyngeal nursing; Oropharyngeal care	口咽护理；口咽部护理
orosomucoid 1; Alpha 1 acid glycoprotein; a-1 acid glycoprotein; α-1 acid glycoprotein; ORM1	血清类黏蛋白1
Orpington Prognostic Scale; OPS	奥平顿预后量表；Orpington预后量表
Orthostatic hypotension; orthostatic hypotension; postural hypotension; Postural hypotension; Orthostatic hypotension (disorder)	体位性低血压；直立性低血压
Orthostatic hypotension due to autonomic dysfunction; Postural hypotension caused by autonomic nerve dysfunction	自主神经功能障碍性体位性低血压；自主神经功能紊乱引起的体位性低血压
Orthostatic syncope	直立性晕厥；直立性虚脱
Orthotic device; orthopedic instrument; orthopaedics instrument; orthosis; Orthotics	矫形器
Osmotherapy; osmotic therapy	渗透疗法

续　表

英文术语	中文术语
Osmotic demyelination; Osmotic demyelination syndrome	渗透性脱髓鞘；渗出性脱髓鞘
osteonectin; SPARC	骨黏连蛋白
Other rehabilitation; other kinds rehabilitation	其他康复
Outcome; Outcomes; Outcomes of stroke; Outcome of stroke; Stroke outcomes; Stroke outcome	结局；疗效；预后；结果
outpatient clinic; outpatient; outpatient serviceclinic; outpatient services; outpatient treatment; outpatient clinics; outpatient department; ambulatory care	门诊；门诊部；医院门诊；门诊医疗
Oxfordshire Community Stroke Project; Oxford Stroke Classification; Bamford classification; OCSP	Oxford 卒中分类
Oxidative stress; Oxidative stress pathway; oxidant stress; oxidation stress; oxidative stress induced; oxidative; reactive oxygen species; oxidative damage; oxidation	氧化应激；氧化性应激；氧化胁迫；氧化损伤；氧化应激反应；氧化应激损伤
Oxidative stress biomarkers of stroke; Oxidative stress biomarker of stroke	脑卒中氧化应激生物标志物
oxidative stress response pathway; oxidative stress pathway; oxidative stress reaction pathway	氧化应激通路；氧化应激反应通路；应激反应通路
Oxidized low-density lipoprotein; Oxidation of low density lipoprotein cholesterol; Oxidation of low density lipoprotein; Oxidation of LDL; LDL-C oxidation; LDL oxidation; Oxidized LDL; Ox-LDL	氧化型低密度脂蛋白；低密度脂蛋白胆固醇氧化；低密度脂蛋白氧化
Oxygen saturation; arterial oxygen saturation	氧饱和度；血氧饱和度；氧饱和(作用)；血氧
P-Selectin; Platelet alpha Granule Membrane Protein; CD62P Antigen; P Selectin	P-选择素
p38 MAPK signaling pathway	p38MAPK信号通路；MAPK信号通路；p38丝裂原活化蛋白激酶(MAPK)信号通路
Pain insensitivity; analgesia	痛觉缺失；疼痛不敏感；痛觉不敏感
Palatal myoclonus; palatal myoclonus; Palatal myoclonus (disorder)	软腭阵挛；腭肌阵挛；腭震颤；腭肌肌阵挛；腭肌痉挛；腭肌肌震颤；腭肌震颤
Palatal weakness; palatal inability; palatal debility	腭部无力；腭部缺陷；腭部不足

英文术语	中文术语
Palinopsia; Visual perseveration; Palinopsia (finding)	视像存留
Palipsychism; psychology; psychological; psychics; psycology; psychological perspective; mentality; psychological knowledge	心理学；心理
Palmitic acid; Hexadecanoic Acid	棕榈酸；软脂酸；十六酸；十六烷酸
paramedian artery infarction symptom; Paraarterial infarction symptoms	旁动脉梗死症状；旁动脉梗塞症状
Paraoxonase 1; Aryldialkylphosphatase; Paraoxonase-1	对氧磷酶1
Paresthesia; Paraesthesia; Paresthesia (finding); Paresthesias; Abnormal sensation; Abnormal sensation (finding)	感觉异常；触觉异常
PARK 7; parkinson disease protein 7; PARK7 protein, human; DJ1 protein, human; protein DJ-1; DJ-1	帕金森病蛋白7
Paroxysmal choreoathetosis; Mount-Reback syndrome; Paroxysmal kinesigenic choreoathetosis; Paroxysmal choreoathetosis (disorder); paroxysmal choreoathetosis	发作性舞蹈手足徐动症；发作性舞蹈样手足徐动；阵发性舞蹈手足徐动症；发作性舞蹈-手足徐动症；舞蹈手足徐动症(发作性)；舞蹈-手足徐动症(发作性)；舞蹈手足徐动症(阵发性)
Paroxysmal dystonia; paroxysmal dystonia; Paroxysmal dystonia (disorder)	阵发性肌张力障碍；发作性肌张力障碍；突发性张力障碍；肌张力发作性障碍
Paroxysmal vertigo; Paroxysmal vertigo (finding)	阵发性眩晕；发作性眩晕
PARP inhibitors; poly ADP ribose polymerase inhibitors; poly ADP ribose polymerase inhibitor; PARP inhibitor	PARP抑制剂
Partial thromboplastin time; PTT; partial thromboplastic time; partial thromboplastin time test; activated partial thromboplastin time	部分凝血活酶时间；部分凝血酶原时间；部分促凝血酶原激酶时间；部分凝血酶时间；部分促凝血酶原时间
Passive joint motion; joints passive movement	关节被动活动
passive smoking; Environmental tobacco smoke; avoid passive tobacco smoke; passive tobacco smoke	被动吸烟；环境烟草烟气；环境烟气；环境香烟烟雾；环境烟草烟雾
pathogenesis; mechanism ; pathogenetic mechanism ; pathological mechanism ; pathologic mechanism ; pathogenic mechanisms ; pathogenesis mechanism ; Nosogenesis	发病机制

续　表

英文术语	中文术语
Pathophysiology of Atherosclerotic cerebrovascular disease; physiopathology of atherosclerotic cerebrovascular disease; pathological physiology of atherosclerotic cerebrovascular disease; pathology of atherosclerotic cerebrovascular disease; pathology and physiology of atherosclerotic cerebrovascular disease	动脉粥样硬化性脑血管病的病理生理学
Patient education; patients education; healthy education; medication education	患者教育；患方教育；用药教育；患者宣教；病人用药指导
Pendular nystagmus; pendular nystagmus; Pendular nystagmus (disorder)	钟摆样眼球震颤；摆动性眼球震颤；钟摆样眼震；摆动性眼振；钟摆式眼球震颤
Pentobarbital; pentobarbital	戊巴比妥；苯巴比妥钠；苯巴比妥；戊巴比妥钠
Perfusion weighted magnetic resonance imaging; Perfusion Magnetic Resonance Imaging; Perfusion weighted MRI; PWI	灌注加权磁共振成像
Pericentral scotoma; pericentral scotoma; Pericentral scotoma (finding)	旁中心暗点；中心周围暗点；中心外周暗点
Peripheral visual field constriction with 10-20 degrees central field preserved; Reduced peripheral vision and retained 10-20 degrees central vision	周边视野缩小且保留 10-20 度中心视野；周边视野狭窄，中央视野保留 10 - 20 度
Peripheral visual field constriction with 20-30 degrees central field preserved; Reduced peripheral vision and retained 20-30 degree central vision	周边视野缩小且保留 20-30 度中心视野；周边视野狭窄，中央视野保留 20 - 30 度
Peripheral visual field constriction with 30-40 degrees central field preserved; Reduced peripheral vision and retained 30-40 degree central vision	周边视野缩小且保留 30-40 度中心视野；周边视野狭窄，中央视野保留 30 - 40 度
Peripheral visual field constriction with 40-50 degrees central field preserved; Reduced peripheral vision and retained 40-50 degree central vision	周边视野缩小且保留 40-50 度中心视野；周边视野狭窄，中央视野保留 40 - 50 度
Peripheral visual field constriction with >50 degrees central field preserved; Narrow peripheral vision and retain > 50 degree central vision	周边视野缩小且保留 >50 度中心视野；周边视野狭窄，中央视野保持 > 50 度
Peripheral visual field constriction with<10 degrees central field preserved; Reduced peripheral vision and retained < 10 degree central vision	周边视野缩小且保留 <10 度中心视野；周边视野狭窄，中央视野保留 < 10°

英文术语	中文术语
Peripheral visual field loss; Loss of peripheral vision; vision of peripheral field loss	周边视野缺损；周边视野丢失；周边视野缺失；周边视野损失
Personal ability evaluation; Personal ability assessment	个人能力评价；个人能力评估
Personal care attendants; Personal care staff; Personal care service personnel; Personal care service staff; Personal care attendant	个人护理服务人员；个人护理服务员；个护服务员
Personality changes; Change in personality; Change in personality (disorder)	性格改变；人格改变；性格转变
personnel; staff; personals; personnel and staff; staffs	人员；全体人员；成员
Pharynx and vocal cord weakness; vocal cord and pharyngeal weakness	咽喉和声带无力；咽和声带无力
Phase Contrast MRA; PC MRA	相位对比MRA
Phenylpropanolamine; phenylpropylamine alcohol	苯丙醇胺；去甲麻黄碱
phosphatidylinositol 3-kinase-Akt signaling pathway; PI3K-Akt signaling pathway	磷脂酰肌醇3-激酶-蛋白激酶B信号通路
Physiatrist; Physiotherapist	理疗师；物理治疗医师
Physical biomarkers of stroke; Physical biomarker of stroke; Physical markers of stroke; Physical marker of stroke	脑卒中的物理生物标志物
Physical Examination; Physical examinations; physical examination	查体；健康查体；体格检查；体格检查
physical therapist; physiotherapist; physiotherapists ; Physical Therapist; Physical and Occupational Therapists	物理治疗师；理疗师；理疗学家
Physical therapy; Physical therapy procedure; Physiotherapy; physical therapy; physiotherapy	理疗；物理治疗；物理疗法
Physicians; physician; physician internist; internists; internist	内科医生；医师；临床医师；住院医师；医者；医务人员；内科医师；全科医生
Pioglitazone	吡格列酮；盐酸吡格列酮；匹格列酮；吡咯列酮
Piracetam	吡拉西坦；吡烷酮醋胺；酰胺吡酮；脑复康
Plasminogen activator inhibitor 1; Plasminogen activator inhibitor-1; PAI 1; PAI-1; PAI1	纤溶酶原激活物抑制物1

续　表

英文术语	中文术语
Platelet activating factor; PAF	血小板活化因子；血小板激活因子；血小板活性因子；血小板活化分子；血小板活化功能
Platelet count; Platelet; platelet; Thrombocyte; blood platelet; Platelet count - finding	血小板计数；血小板
platelet derived growth factor a; platelet-derived growth factor-alpha; platelet-derived growth factor-a; PDGFA	血小板衍生生长因子a
Platelet derived hemostasis regulated genes; Platelet-derived hemostasis regulated genes in atherosclerotic stroke	血小板源性止血调节基因
Platelet factor 4; gamma-Thromboglobulin; Platelet factor Ⅳ; Chemokine CXCL4; Factor Ⅳ; PF4	血小板因子4
Platelet glycoprotein Ⅱ b of Ⅱ b Ⅲ a complex; Platelet glycoprotein Ⅱ b of Ⅱ b/ Ⅲ a complex; ITGA2B	Ⅱ b Ⅲ a复合物的血小板糖蛋白 Ⅱ b
Platelet glycoprotein Ⅲ a of Ⅱ b Ⅲ a complex; Platelet glycoprotein Ⅲ a of Ⅱ b/ Ⅲ a complex; ITGB3	Ⅱ b Ⅲ a复合物的血小板糖蛋白 Ⅲ a
Pneumonia; Pneumonitis; pneumonia; Pneumonitis (disorder); Pneumonia (disorder)	肺炎
Poly ADP ribose polymerase 1; PARP1 Protein; PARP1	聚ADP核糖聚合酶1；聚ADP核糖聚合酶1蛋白
Poly ADP ribose polymerase activation; Poly [ADP-ribose] polymerase; Poly (ADP-ribose) polymerase; PARP activation; PARP	多聚ADP核糖聚合酶活化；多聚(ADP-核糖)聚合酶
polyamine glutamate antagonist; polyamine glutamate antagonists; polyamine glutamate inhibitor	多胺谷氨酸拮抗剂
Polyamine metabolites	多胺类代谢产物
Polyarteritis nodosa; polyarteritis nodosa; polyarteritis nodusa; POLYARTERITIS NODOSA; Periarteritis nodosa; PAN - Polyarteritis nodosa; Polyarteritis nodosa (disorder)	结节性多动脉炎；结节性多发性动脉炎；结节性动脉周围炎；多动脉炎
Polyunsaturated fatty acid; PUFA	多不饱和脂肪酸
Pontine artery	桥脑动脉
Pontine infarct symptom; Symptoms of pontine infarction; Symptom of pontine infarction; Pontine infarct symptoms	桥脑梗死症状；桥脑梗塞症状
position; body position; body posture; Position; Posture; posture	体位；姿势

英文术语	中文术语
position management; posture managing; posture management; position control; postural management; body position management	体位管理
position placement; body position; body placement; postural placement; posture placement	体位摆放；体位安置
Post seizure weakness	癫痫发作后乏力；发作后虚弱；发作后无力
Post stroke comorbidity; Post stroke comorbidities	卒中后合并症；脑卒中后合并症
Post stroke dementia; Post stroke cognitive impairment; PSD	卒中后痴呆；脑卒中后痴呆
Post stroke depression; ischemic post-stroke depression; post ischemic stroke depression	卒中后抑郁；中风后抑郁；缺血性脑卒中后抑郁；缺血性中风后抑郁
Posterior cerebral artery; Posterior cerebral arteries; PCAs; PCA; posterior cerebral artery	大脑后动脉
Posterior cerebral artery infarction syndrome; syndromes of posterior cerebral artery infarction; syndrome of posterior cerebral artery infarction; Posterior cerebral artery infarction symptom; PCA infarction symptom	大脑后动脉梗死综合征
Posterior choroidal artery; Posterior choroidal arteries; PChAs; PChA	脉络膜后动脉
Posterior Choroidal artery infarction symptom; Dorsal thalamic infarction; PChA infarction symptom	脉络膜后动脉梗死症状；后脉络膜动脉梗死症状；后脉络膜动脉梗塞症状
Posterior communicating artery; Posterior communicating arteries; PCoAs; PCoA; posterior communicating artery	后交通动脉
Posterior inferior cerebellar artery; PICA	小脑后下动脉
Posterior inferior cerebellar artery embolism; Posterior inferior cerebellar artery embolization; Posterior inferior cerebellar artery thromboembolism; posterior inferior cerebellar arteries embolism; posterior inferior cerebellar artery embolism	小脑后下动脉栓塞；小脑后下动脉血栓栓塞
Posterior inferior cerebellar artery infarction symptom; PICA infarction symptom	小脑后下动脉梗死症状；小脑后下动脉梗塞症状
Poststroke hyperglycemia; post stroke hyperglycemia	卒中后高血糖；卒中后血糖高

续　表

英文术语	中文术语
Poststroke Osteoporosis; Post-stroke osteoporosis; Post-stroke osteoporotic; Post-stroke bone rarefaction; Post-stroke bone osteoporosis; Post-stroke osteopenia; Post-stroke osteoporotic fracture	卒中后骨质疏松；脑卒中后骨质疏松
Postural Assessment Scale for Stroke Patients; PASS	脑卒中患者体位评估量表
Postural hypotension with compensatory tachycardia	体位性低血压伴代偿性心动过速
Postural tremor; postural tremor; Orthostatic tremor; Orthostatic tremor (finding)	姿势性震颤；体位性震颤；直立性震颤
Potential for further improvement; Potential for further improve	进一步改善的可能性；进一步改善的潜力
Poultry; fowl; chicken; avian; domestic fowls; domestic fowl	家禽；禽；鸡；畜禽；肉鸡；鸡肉；鸡类
PPAR agonist	PPAR 激动剂
PPAR-a agonist; PPAR alpha agonist; PPAR-alpha agonist; PPAR a agonist; PPARA agonist	PPAR - α 激动剂
PPAR-g agonist; PPAR gama agonist; PPAR-gama agonist; PPAR g agonist; PPARG agonist	PPAR-g 激动剂
Pravastatin	普伐他汀；匹伐他汀
Prediabetes; Prediabetes (finding); Prediabetic nonclinical diabetes	糖尿病前期；前驱糖尿病；糖尿病前驱期
pressure sore rehabilitation nursing; Rehabilitation nursing of pressure ulcer	压疮康复护理；褥疮康复护理
Prestroke comorbidity; Pre stroke comorbidities; Pre-stroke comorbidities; Prestroke comorbidities; Pre-stroke comorbidity; Pre stroke comorbidity	卒中前合并症
Prevention; prophylaxis; Prophylaxis; prevention	预防；防治；防止
Prevention of epileptic seizures; Seizure Prophylaxis; Prevention of seizures; Prevention of epileptic seizure	预防痫性发作；痫性发作预防
Prevention of Falls; falling prevention; preventing falling; tumbling prevention; preventive falling; tumbles prevention; fall prevention; prevention of tumble	预防跌倒；防跌倒
previous history; historical information; past medical history; anamnesis; prior history; previous medical history	既往史；过去病史；既往病史

英文术语	中文术语
Primary hypercholesterolemia; Primary hypercholesterolaemia; Primary hypercholesterolemia (disorder)	原发性高胆固醇血症
Primary hypertriglyceridemia; Primary hypertriglyceridaemia; Primary hypertriglyceridemia (disorder)	原发性高甘油三酯血症
Primary prevention of atherosclerotic cerebrovascular disease; Primary atherosclerotic cerebrovascular disease prevention; prevent first stroke	动脉粥样硬化性脑血管病的一级预防；动脉粥样硬化性脑血管病的初级预防；脑血管病的一级预防
Primary rehabilitation; first grade rehabilitation; primary recovery	一级康复
Primary rehabilitation training; Primary rehabilitation exercise; Primary rehabilitative training; Primary rehabilitation therapy; Primary rehabilitation treatment	一级康复训练
Primary stroke center; Stroke Care Unit; PSC; SCU	初级卒中中心
Prior stroke; Old cerebrovascular accident; Old stroke; Old CVA	既往卒中；陈旧性脑血管意外
Processed meat	加工肉制品；预处理肉；加工肉；熟肉制品；热加工肉；加工肉类
Procoagulants; procoagulation mediator; Procoagulant	凝血激活物；促凝介质
Professional nursing institutions; SNFs; Skilled Nursing Facilities; specialized nursing institutions	专业护理机构
Progressive cerebellar ataxia; progressive cerebellar ataxia; Progressive cerebellar ataxia (disorder)	进行性小脑共济失调；进行性小脑性共济失调
Progressive choreoathetosis; Progressive dance moves	进行性舞蹈手足徐动症；进行性舞蹈样手足徐动；渐进性舞蹈手足徐动
Progressive gait ataxia	进行性共济失调
Progressive ptosis; incremental ptosis	进行性上睑下垂；渐进性上睑下垂
Progressive truncal ataxia	进行性躯干共济失调
Progressive visual field defects; Lack of progressive vision	进行性视野缺损；渐进性视野缺损；渐进性视野缺失；进行性视野缺失
Projectile vomiting; Projectile vomiting (disorder); projectile charge vomiting; projectile vomiting	喷射性呕吐；喷射状呕吐
proprioceptive neuromuscular facilitaion; PNF	本体感觉神经肌肉促进技术

续　表

英文术语	中文术语
Prosopagnosia; prosopagnosia; Agnosia for faces; Prosopagnosia (finding)	面容失认；面容失认症；面孔失认症；面部失认；脸盲症；人面失认症；面孔遗忘症
prostaglandin endoperoxide synthase 2; cyclooxygenase-2; PTGS2	前列腺素内过氧化物合酶2；前列腺素内过氧化物合成酶2
Prostanoids; prostaglandin; prostaglandins; lipo-prostaglandin; prostaglandin e2; prostacyclin	前列腺烷酸类；前列腺素；前列腺素类
Protanomaly; protanomalia	红色弱视；红色弱
Protanopia; red blindness	红色盲；第一原色盲；甲型色盲
Protein aggregates; protein aggregation; protein aggresome; protein aggregate	蛋白聚体；蛋白聚集；蛋白质聚集体；蛋白沉积
Protein C	蛋白C
Protein carbonyls	蛋白羰基；脂质过氧化(MDA)；蛋白质羰基化
Protein S	蛋白S
Proteinase activated receptor 1; PAR-1; PAR1	蛋白酶激活受体1
Proteomics biomarkers of stroke	脑卒中的蛋白质组学生物标志物
Prothrombin; Factor II; Coagulation factor II; Thrombinogen	凝血酶原；凝血因子Ⅱ；因子Ⅱ
Prothrombin fragment 1; Prothrombin fragment-1	凝血酶原片段1
Prothrombin fragment 2; Prothrombin fragment-2	凝血酶原片段2
Prothrombin gene mutation; Prothrombin G20210 mutation	凝血酶原基因突变；凝血酶原G20210突变
Prothrombin time; PT; proth time prothrombin time; blood prothrombin time; thrombinogen time; prothrombin time; thromboplastin time; thrombin time	凝血酶原时间；血浆凝血酶原时间；前凝血酶时间；血浆凝血酶原时间测定
Proton magnetic resonance spectroscopy image; Proton Magnetic Resonance Spectroscopy; H-MRS image	质子磁共振波谱图像
prudent diet; Careful diet	谨慎饮食；精细饮食；细致饮食
Pseudobulbar palsy; pseudobulbar paralysis; Supranuclear paralysis; pseudobulbar palsy; Pseudobulbar paralysis; Supranuclear paralysis (disorder); Pseudobulbar palsy (disorder)	假性球麻痹；假性延髓性麻痹；假性延髓麻痹；假延髓性麻痹；假性麻痹(延髓性)；延髓性假性麻痹

英文术语	中文术语
Pseudoradicular sensory deficit; Pseudoradicular sensory disturbance; Pseudoradicular sensation disorders; Pseudoradicular sensory disorder; Pseudoradicular sensory distrubance; Pseudoradicular esthesic disorder; Pseudoradicular sensation disturbance	假性神经根感觉障碍；假性神经根感觉减退；假性神经根感觉缺失；假性神经根感觉缺损
Pseudoseizure with tonic spasm; Pseudoseizure with tetanic spasm; Pseudoseizure with ankylosing spasm	假性发作伴强直性痉挛；假性发作伴紧张性痉挛
Pseudoxanthoma elasticum; pseudoxanthoma elasticum; PXE; Nevus elasticus; Naevus elasticus; Elastic naevus; Elastic nevus; Nevus elasticus (disorder); PXE - Pseudoxanthoma elasticum; Pseudoxanthoma elasticum (disorder)	弹性纤维假黄瘤；弹性假黄色瘤；弹性假黄瘤；弹力纤维假黄瘤；弹性痣；弹性假黄瘤病
Pseudoxanthoma elasticum autosomal dominant form; Pseudoxanthoma elasticum AD form	弹性假黄瘤常染色体显性形态
Pseudoxanthoma elasticum autosomal recessive form; Pseudoxanthoma elasticum AR form	弹性假黄瘤常染色体隐性形态
psychological assessment; psychological evaluation; emotional appraisal; emotion evaluation; emotional evaluation; emotion appraisal	心理评估；情感评价；情感评估；情绪评价
psychological nursing; mental nursing	心理干预；心理护理；心理护理干预；心理行为护理；心理护理学
Psychological therapy; psychotherapy; psychological treatment; psychological intervention; psychology therapy; psychology treatment; therapy psychotherapy	心理治疗；心理疗法
Psychologists; psychologist	心理医师；心理学家
Ptosis; ptosis; blepharoptosis; ptosis of eyelid; Drooping upper eyelid; Ptosis of eyelid; Blepharoptosis; Eyelid ptosis; Ptosis eyelid; Drooping eyelid; Droopy eyelid; Ptosis of eyelid (disorder)	上睑下垂；上胞下垂；睑下垂；(上)睑下垂；眼睑下垂；眼睑下垂；上眼睑下垂
public health education; pubic health education	公共健康教育；公众健康教育；公共卫生教育；民众卫生教育；民众健康教育

续　表

英文术语	中文术语
Pulmonary embolism; PE; pulmonary embolism; Pulmonary Embolism; Pulmonary thrombosis; Pulmonary thrombosis (disorder); Pulmonary infarction; Pulmonary infarct; Pulmonary infarction (disorder); Pulmonary artery thrombosis; Pulmonary arterial thrombosis; Pulmonary artery thrombosis (disorder); PE - Pulmonary embolism; Pulmonary embolism (disorder); Pulmonary thromboembolism; PE - Pulmonary thromboembolism; PTE - Pulmonary thromboembolism; Pulmonary thromboembolism (disorder)	肺栓塞；肺动脉栓塞；肺动脉梗塞；肺动脉血栓；肺血栓；肺血栓栓塞症；肺血栓栓塞
Pulsatile tinnitus; pulsatile tinnitus; Tinnitus of vascular origin; Vascular tinnitus; Tinnitus of vascular origin (disorder)	搏动性耳鸣；血管源性耳鸣；血管性耳鸣；跳动性耳鸣
Pulse rate; pulse rate	脉率；脉搏率
pupillary light reflex; pupil light reflex	瞳孔对光反射；对光反射；瞳孔对光反应
Pure motor hemiparesis; Simple motor hemiplegia; Pure motor hemiplegia; Simple motor hemiparesis; PMH	纯运动性轻偏瘫；纯运动偏瘫；纯运动轻偏瘫；单纯运动性半身不遂；单纯运动性偏瘫
Pure sensory stroke; Simple sensory stroke	纯感觉性卒中；单纯感觉性卒中；纯感觉性中风
push method; Push-pull therapy; push brace therapy; Push-pull treatment; push brace treatment	推举法；推撑疗法
Race; Race-ethnic groups; race relations; Race-ethnic; Ethnicity; Ethnic	种族；民族；人种
Radiation vasculopathy; Radioactive vascular disease	放射性血管病；放射性血管病变
Ramipril	雷米普利；瑞泰；拉米普利；雷米普利片
Raymond syndrome	Raymond综合征；Raymond征；雷蒙德综合征
Reactive nitrogen species generation; RNS generation; Reactive nitrogen species formation	活性氮生成；反应性氮物种生成
Reactive oxygen species generation; Reactive oxygen species; ROS generation; ROS	活性氧生成；活性氧簇生成；活性氧基团
Rebleeding	破裂再出血；复发出血；颅内动脉瘤再破裂

英文术语	中文术语
Red meat intake; Low red meat consumption	红肉摄入量
Red-green dyschromatopsia; Red-green disturbance	红绿色觉障碍
Reduced fat milk; low-fat milk	低脂牛奶
Rehabilitation; Rehabilitation therapy; Rehabilitation care; rehabilitation	康复；康复疗法；康复护理
rehabilitation assessment; rehabilitation evaluation; rehabilitation evaluation and assessment	康复评价；康复评估；康复评定；康复评定学；康复测评；康复疗效评估；康复疗法评定学
rehabilitation centre; rehabilitation center; restored to health center; health recovery center; health center; rehablitation center	康复中心
Rehabilitation demand evaluation; rehabilitation needs evaluation; rehabilitation demand assessment; rehabilitation needs assessment	康复需求评价；康复需求评估
Rehabilitation Department; rehabilitation medicine department; rehabilitation medical department; rehabilitation medicine	康复医学科；康复科
rehabilitation equipment; rehab equip; rehabilitation devices; rehabilitation device	康复设备；康复器械；康复仪器；康复器具；康复运动器材
rehabilitation management; recovery management; rehabilitation administration	康复管理；康复治疗；康复护理；疗养管理
Rehabilitation Nurses; rehabilitative nurse; rehabilitative nurses; rehabilitation nurse	康复护士；康复护理；康复专科护士
Rehabilitation nursing of hemiplegia; Hemiplegia rehabilitation nursing care; Hemiplegia rehabilitation nurse; Hemiplegia rehabilitation care; Hemiplegia rehabilitation medical attendance; hemiplegic rehabilitation nursing	偏瘫康复护理；偏瘫康复训练
rehabilitation of aphasia; Aphasia rehabilitation; aphasia	语言障碍康复；失语症康复
Rehabilitation of cognitive impairment; Rehabilitation of cognitive disorder; Rehabilitation of cognitive disorders; Rehabilitation of cognition disorder; rehabilitation of cognitive impairment	认知障碍康复；认知功能康复
Rehabilitation of dysarthria; Rehabilitation of dysarthrosis; Rehabilitation of anarthria	构音障碍康复；构音不良康复；构音困难康复
Rehabilitation of dysuria; Rehabilitation of urinary and fecal disorders	尿便障碍康复；排尿困难的康复

续　表

英文术语	中文术语
Rehabilitation of emotional disorders; Rehabilitation of emotional handicap; recovery of emotional handicap; recovery of emotional disorders	情绪障碍康复；情感障碍康复
Rehabilitation of language and communication disorders	语言和交流障碍康复；语言和沟通障碍的康复
Rehabilitation of motor dysfunction; Rehabilitation of movement disorders; Rehabilitation of motor function disorders; Rehabilitation of motor functional deficits; Rehabilitation of movement dysfunction; Rehabilitation of motor function disorder; Rehabilitation of motor functional disorder	运动功能障碍康复；运动障碍康复
rehabilitation system	康复体系；康复系统；康复训练系统
rehabilitation therapist; Reconstruction therapist; Recreation Therapists	康复治疗师；娱乐治疗师；康复师；重建治疗师
rehabilitation wards; rehabilitation ward	康复病房；康复病区
Remacemide	瑞马西胺
Remote stroke medicine	远程卒中医疗；远程卒中
Renal function tests; Kidney function tests; Renal function study; Renal function test	肾功能检查；肾功能；肾功能检验；肾功能试验
Reorganization memory method; Reorganization method	重新组织记忆法；重新组织法
Repeated saliva swallowing examination	反复唾液吞咽检查；反复唾液吞咽检测
Reperfusion therapy; reperfusion treatment; reperfusion; reperfusion strategies	再灌注治疗；再灌注疗法；灌注治疗
Repetitive transcranial magnetic stimulatio; rTMS	重复经颅磁刺激
Repinotan	雷皮诺坦
respiration training; respiratory functional training; breath training; respiratory function exercise; breath instruction; breath exercise; breathing exercise	呼吸训练；呼吸运动
respiratory management; airway management; respiratory tract management; respiratory tract care; respiratory tract; respiratory tract control; supervision of respiratory tract; management of airway	呼吸道管理；呼吸管理；呼吸道护理
Respiratory rate; respiratory frequency; respiratory rates; breath frequency	呼吸频率；呼吸速率；呼吸率；呼吸强度

续　表

英文术语	中文术语
Resting tremor; Static tremor; Static tremor (finding); Rest tremor; resting tremor; Resting tremor (finding)	静止性震颤；休息性震颤
Restoration memory method; recalling memory method; refreshing memory method; retrieving memory method; memory recovery method	恢复记忆法；恢复记忆方法
Reteplase	瑞替普酶；瑞替辅酶；雷特普酶
Retinal vasculitis; retinal vasculitis; Retinal vasculitis (disorder)	视网膜血管炎；视网膜血管周围炎；视网膜脉管炎
retinoic acid signaling pathway; RA signaling pathway	维甲酸信号通路
Retinol; Vitamin A; retinol; vitamin A	视黄醇；维生素A
Retrocollis	颈后倾
Return to Driving; resume driving; Recover driving	恢复驾驶；回归驾驶；重新驾驶
Return to Work; reentry	重返工作；恢复工作；复职；返岗；再就业
ribonuclease 2; ribonuclease-2; RNASE2	核糖核酸酶2
Rice intake; Low rice consumption	大米摄入量
Right carotid artery atherosclerosis; Atherosclerosis of right carotid artery; Right carotid artery atherosclerosis (disorder); Atherosclerosis of right carotid artery (disorder)	右颈动脉粥样硬化；右颈动脉粥样硬化斑块；右颈动脉硬化
Right-left disorientation; Left-right confusion; Right-left disorientation (finding)	左右失认；左-右混乱；左右定向障碍
Ring scotoma; ring scotoma; Ring scotoma (finding)	环形暗点；环状暗点
ring up; phone; dial; telephone; call; talking on the phone	打电话
Risk assessment of deep vein thrombosis; Risk evaluation of deep vein thrombosis; Risk evaluation of deep venous thrombosis; Risk assessment of deep venous thrombosis	深静脉血栓形成风险评价；深静脉血栓危险性评估；深静脉血栓形成风险评估
Risk factor; Risk factors of stroke; Risk factor of stroke; Stroke risk factors; Stroke risk factor; Risk of stroke; Risk factors	危险因素；病因；风险因素；影响因素；风险因子；高危因素；危险因子
Risk factor reduction; Reduced risk factors	降低风险因素；风险因素降低；危险因素降低；风险因素减少；危险因素减少
Rivaroxaban; shaaban	利伐沙班；利伐他班

续　表

英文术语	中文术语
Rivermead ADL assessment	Rivermead ADL 评定法
Rivermead Behavioral Inattention Test; RBIT	Rivermead行为注意力测试
Rivermead Mobility Index; RMI	Rivermead 活动指数
Rivermead Motor Assessment	Rivermead 运动评估
Robotic and Electromechanics-Assisted Training Devices; Robot and electromechanical auxiliary training equipment	机器人和机电辅助训练设备；机器人及机电辅助训练设备
Rood sensorimotor apporoach; Rood Sensory Exercise Therapy	Rood感觉运动治疗方法；Rood感觉运动疗法；Rood法
Rosiglitazone	罗格列酮；马来酸罗格列酮；罗格列酮钠；盐酸罗格列酮
Rotary nystagmus; Rotatory nystagmus; Rotary nystagmus (disorder)	旋转性眼球震颤；旋转眼球震颤；旋转眼震；旋转性眼震
Routine exercise; convention exercise; common practice exercise; method routine exercise; normality exercise; ordinary discontinuity practice exercise; customary practice exercise	常规锻炼；常规运动；日常锻炼；日常运动
rt-PA; Tissue Plasminogen Activator; Tissue-type plasminogene activator; Tissue type plasminogene activator; Alteplase; Activase	阿替普酶
Rubral tremor; Abdominal tremor	红核震颤；腹部震颤
S100 beta; S100 Calcium Binding Protein beta; S100-beta; S100B	S100β；S100 钙结合蛋白β
S100 calcium binding protein A12; s100A12	S100 钙结合蛋白 A12
S100 calcium binding proteins A9; S100A9	S100 钙结合蛋白 A9
S100 calcium binding proteins P; S100P	S100 钙结合蛋白 P
Salt; table salt; dairy salt; daily salt; celery salt; common salt; butter salt; iodized salt	食盐；盐；盐分；盐含量
SATIS Stroke	SATIS卒中
Saturated fatty acid; Saturated fats; Saturated fat; Fatty acids; Fatty acid; Saturated fatty acids intake; Saturated fatty acids; Saturated fat intake; Saturated fat diet; fatty acid	饱和脂肪酸；脂肪酸；游离脂肪酸；饱和脂肪酸含量；一元脂肪酸；一元饱和脂肪酸；饱和脂肪；有机酸
Scales; Scoring grading test and classification systems; Classification systems; Scoring systems; Stroke scale; Grading; Scale; scale	量表

英文术语	中文术语
Scandinavian stroke scale; SSS	斯堪得维亚脑卒中量表；Scandinavian 脑卒中量表评分
scapula mobilization; Scapular loosening	肩胛骨松动术
Scavenger receptor; Macrophage Scavenger Receptors; Macrophage Scavenger Receptor; Acetyl LDL Receptors; Acetyl LDL Receptor	清道夫受体；巨噬细胞清道夫受体；乙酰基低密度脂蛋白受体
Scavenger receptor class B member 1; CD36 protein; SR-BI; SRB1; CD36 antigen-like 1; SR-BI Receptor; SR-BI Protein; CD-36 protein; CD36 Antigens	清道夫受体B类成员1；Cd36类抗原1；B组1型清道夫受体；CD36蛋白；CD36抗原
Scavenger Receptors, Class A; Class A Scavenger Receptors; SR-A Proteins	清道夫受体，A类；A类清道夫受体
Schuellapha-sic stimulation approach	许尔失语症刺激疗法；Schuell 刺激法
Scintillating scotoma; Flittering scotoma; Scintillating scotoma (finding)	闪光性暗点；闪烁的暗点；(偏头痛)闪烁幻象；闪光性幻象
Scotoma; Blind spot; blind spot; scotoma; SCOTOMA; Visual field scotoma; Visual field scotoma (finding)	暗点；盲点
Screening for diabetic mellitus; Screenung for DM	糖尿病筛查
Screening for Self Medication Safety Post Stroke Scale; S-5	脑卒中后自我用药安全量表筛查
Screening for sleep apnea; Sleep apnea screening	睡眠呼吸暂停筛查；筛查为睡眠呼吸暂停
Secondary hypercholesterolemia; Secondary hypercholesterolaemia; Secondary hypercholesterolemia (disorder)	继发性高胆固醇血症；继发性血胆脂醇过多
Secondary hyperlipidemia; Secondary hyperlipidaemia; Exogenous hyperlipidemia; Exogenous hyperlipidaemia; Exogenous hyperlipaemia; Exogenous hyperlipemia; Exogenous hyperlipidemia (disorder); Secondary hyperlipidemia (disorder)	继发性高脂血症；外源性高脂血症；继发性血脂异常
Secondary hypertriglyceridemia; Secondary hypertriglyceridaemia; Secondary hypertriglyceridemia (disorder)	继发性高甘油三酯血症
Secondary prevention of atherosclerotic cerebrovascular disease; Secondary atherosclerotic cerebrovascular disease prevention	动脉粥样硬化性脑血管病二级预防；脑血管病的二级预防
secondary rehabilitation; secondary rehabilitative; second degree rehabilitative; secondary convalescence	二级康复

续　表

英文术语	中文术语
Secondary rehabilitation training; Secondary rehabilitative training; Secondary rehabilitation trained; Secondary rehabilitative trained	二级康复训练
Sedentary lifestyle; Sedentary life style; Sedentary lifestyle (finding); Sedentary lifestyles; physical inactivity; Inactivity	久坐生活方式；静坐生活方式；静态生活方式
Seed oil; Seed oils; seed kernel oil of; nut oil	菜籽油；籽油；种子油；油脂；麻仁油；植物油
Seesaw nystagmus; See-saw nystagmus; See-saw nystagmus (disorder)	跷跷板眼球震颤；跷跷板状眼球震颤；跷跷板式眼震；跷跷板式眼球震颤
Self monitoring of blood pressure; Home self-monitoring of blood pressure; self-monitoring of BP	血压监测；自我监测血压；血压自我监测
Sensorimotor stroke; Mixed sensorimotor stroke; Sensory motor stroke	感觉运动性卒中；感觉运动性脑卒中
Sensory awakening training; sensation awakening training; sensation arousal training; Sensory arousal training	感觉唤醒训练；感觉觉醒训练；感官觉醒训练
sensory function; sensation function; sense function; sensation functions; feeling function; sensory functions; finger feeling	感觉功能；感知功能；感官功能；感觉机能
sensory impairment; Sensory loss; sensory deprivation; sensory disorder	感觉障碍；感知觉缺失；感觉缺失
Septic intracranial venous thrombosis; Infectious intracranial venous thrombosis	化脓性颅内静脉窦血栓形成；感染性颅内静脉栓塞
Serotonin agonist	5-羟色胺受体激动剂；血清素致效剂；塞罗通激动剂
Serum albumin; Albumin; ALB; albumin	白蛋白；清蛋白
Serum amyloid A protein; Serum amyloid A (SAA) proteins; Serum amyloid A (SAA) protein; Serum amyloid A proteins; SAA proteins; SAA protein; SAA	血清淀粉样蛋白A
Serum bilirubin; Bilirubin; hematoidin; bilirubin	血清胆红素；血清总胆红素；血总胆红素；血清结合胆红素
serum lipid test; Serum lipid profile	血脂检测；血脂试验
Sexual Function; erectile function; sex function; sexual ability; sexual functions; sexual functional; sexual activity	性功能；性机能；性功能状态
shopping; buy things; go shopping	购物；采购；买东西

续 表

英文术语	中文术语
shoulder joints support; Shoulder support; shoulder joint support; scapulohumeral articulation support; articulatio humeri support; glenohumeral joint support	肩关节支撑
Shoulder pain; Pain of shoulder; shoulder pain; Shoulder pain (finding); Pain in shoulder; Shoulder region pain	肩痛；肩疼痛；肩部疼痛
Shwartz Index	史华兹指数；Shwartz 指数
Sickle cell disease; SCD; Sickle cell syndrome; Sickle cell anemia; Sickle cell anaemia	镰状细胞血症；镰状细胞病；镰状细胞贫血
Silent transient hemiparesis; Symptomless temporary hemiplegia	无症状短暂性偏瘫；无症状暂时性偏瘫
Simultanagnosia; simultagnosia	综合性失认
Simvastatin	辛伐他汀；辛伐他汀片；忆辛
Single gene disorders associated with stroke; Stroke-related single-gene diseases	与卒中相关的单基因疾病；与脑卒中相关的单基因障碍
Single-phase CTA; Single phase CTA; spCTA; sCTA	单相CTA
Sitting balance training; Sitting balance train; Sitting balance exercise	坐位平衡训练
Six Minute Walk Test; 6MWD; 6MWT	六分钟步行测试
Skew deviation; skew deviation; Skew deviation (disorder)	反向偏斜；(眼球)反侧偏斜；眼球反侧偏斜
Skin Breakdown and Contractures; Skin ruptures and contractures; Skin fracture and contracture; Skin rupturing and contractures; Skin breakup and contracture; Skin disrupt and contractures; Skin crack and contracture; Skin rupture occurred and contractures; Skin rupture and contracture	皮肤破裂和挛缩；皮肤破损和挛缩
Sleep myoclonus	睡眠肌阵挛
Smoking; Tobacco use; Tobacco; exposure to cigarette smoke; Cigarette smoking; cigarette use; nicotiana tabacum; tabacco	吸烟；吸烟行为
Smoking cessation; Cessation of cigarette smoking; quitting smoking; Smoking addiction cession; tobacco use cessation; stopping smoking; smoking-quitting	戒烟；烟草控制；控烟；戒烟行为；戒烟干预；烟草戒断
Sneddon syndrome; Ehrmann Sneddon syndrome	Sneddon综合征

续　表

英文术语	中文术语
Snoring; Snores; Snoring (finding); Habitual snoring; Snorings; snore; snoring; SNORING	鼾症；打鼾；鼻鼾
Social Workers; social worker; social work; public service worker	社工；社会工作者
Soda intake; consumption of Soda	苏打摄入量；苏打摄入
Sodium intake; Low sodium intake; low sodium diet; Sodium	钠盐摄入；钠；钠摄入；钠摄入量；盐摄入量；钠盐
solute carrier family 2 member 1; SLC2A1	溶质载体家族2成员1
Somnolence; Sleepiness; Drowsy; Mental status, drowsy; Sleepy; Drowsiness; Somnolence (sleepiness); Drowsy (finding)	嗜睡状态；倦睡；嗜眠
Soy protein; soybean protein; soy protein; soy protein isolate; soybean proteins; soy proteins	大豆蛋白；大豆蛋白质；大豆分离蛋白
Spasmus nutans; spasmus nutans; nodding spasm; Salaam spasm; Nodding spasm; Salaam spasm (finding); Spasmus nutans (disorder)	点头痉挛；点头状痉挛
Spastic ataxia	痉挛性共济失调
Spastic dysarthria; Spastic dysarthria (finding)	痉挛性构音障碍；痉挛性构语障碍；痉挛型构音障碍
Spatial disorientation; Disorientation as to space; Spatial disorientation (finding)	空间定向力障碍；空间定向障碍
spectral analysis; spectrum analysis; frequency spectrum analysis; frequency analysis	频谱分析；光谱分析；谱分析
Speech apraxia; alexia; Alexia; Word blindness; Optical alexia; Alexia (finding)	失读症；视觉性失读；失读
Speech therapy; language therapy; voice therapy; speech-language therapy; Speech Therapies; therapy by speech therapist	言语治疗；语音治疗；言语矫治；言语训练；言语治疗学；语音训练；语言康复治疗；言语矫正；言语疗法
Speech-language Pathologists; speech pathologist	语言障碍矫正师；言语病理学家；语言病理学家
Spermine oxidase; SMO	精胺氧化酶
Sphincter of Oddi dysfunction; sphincter functional disturbance ; sphincter disfunction; sphincter disturbance; Sphincter dysfunction; Sphincter incontinence	Oddi括约肌功能障碍；括约肌功能障碍
Spinach; spinacia; spinage; spinaches	菠菜；圆叶菠菜；尖叶菠菜

续　表

英文术语	中文术语
Spinal myoclonus; Spinal cord myoclonus; Spinal cord myoclonus (disorder)	脊髓肌阵挛；脊髓性肌阵挛
sport; Exercise; Physical activity; sports; motion; exercise; movement; athletic	运动；锻炼；体育锻炼；运动训练；运动锻炼
stairs-climbing; stair ascend and descent; climbing up and down stairs; stairs climbing and descending; up and down stairs; stair climbing; walking up and down stairs	上下楼梯；爬楼梯
standing balance; vertical balance; upright balance	立位平衡；站立平衡
Staphylokinase	葡萄球菌激酶；葡激酶
Statin; 3-hydroxy 3-methylglutaryl coenzyme A reductase inhibitor; 3-hydroxy-3-methylglutaryl-coenzyme A reductase inhibitor; HMG-CoA reductase inhibitors; Statins	他汀类药物；他汀；他汀类药物类药物；他汀药
Statin therapy	他汀治疗；他汀类药物治疗；他汀类药物
Stay away from alcoholic drinks; Mild drinking; slight drinking	戒酒；少量饮酒
Stearic acid; octadecanoic acid; stearinic acid; Cetylacetic Acid; Cetylacetic Acid Stearic Acid	硬脂酸；十八酸；十八烷酸；粉状硬脂酸；三压硬脂酸；脂蜡酸
Stent-based thrombectomy; Endovascular thrombectomy; Stent retriever thrombectomy	支架取栓术；支架血栓切除术
Steroid; steroid	类固醇；甾族化合物
Stop Stroke Study TOAST; SSS-TOAST	改良TOAST分型；TOAST停止中风研究；TOAST阻止卒中研究
Streptokinase; Streptodecase; Distreptase; Kabikinase; Kabivitrum; Streptase; Avelizin; Awelysin; Celiase; streptokinase	链激酶
Stroke Activity Scale; SAS	脑卒中活动量表
Stroke Adapted Sickness Impact Profile; SA-SIP30; SA-SIP	卒中适应疾病影响分布
Stroke Aphasic Depression Questionnaire; SADQ-21; SADQ-10; SADQ-H; SADQ	脑卒中双相抑郁问卷
Stroke Arm Ladder	卒中臂梯
Stroke center	卒中中心；脑卒中中心；脑中风中心
Stroke Impact Scale; SIS 3.0; SIS 2.0; SIS-16; SIS	脑卒中影响量表

续 表

英文术语	中文术语
Stroke recurrence; Stroke recurrent	卒中复发；复发性脑卒中；再发脑卒中；脑卒中复发；再发卒中；再发脑梗死；复发性脑梗死
Stroke Specific Quality Of Life scale; SS-QOL	卒中特异性生活质量量表
stroke unit; stroke units ; apoplexia unit; apoplexy unit	卒中单元；脑卒中单元；中风单元；脑卒中病房；卒中单元病房
Stupor; lethargy; lethargic sleep; Stupor (finding)	昏睡；昏呆；昏沉；木僵
Subdural hemorrhage; Subdural intracranial hemorrhages; Subdural intracranial hemorrhage; Subdural haemorrhages; Subdural haemorrhage; Subdural hemorrhages; Subdural Hematoma; Subdural bleeding; SAH; subdural hemorrhage; Hemorrhage into subdural space of spine; Haemorrhage into subdural space of spine; Hemorrhage into subdural space of spine (disorder); Subdural intracranial haemorrhage; Subdural intracranial hemorrhage (disorder); Subdural hemorrhage (disorder)	硬膜下出血；硬脑膜下出血；脊柱硬膜下出血
Subsequent herniation; Secondary hernia	继发脑疝；随后的疝气；后续疝
Subthalamus nucleus infarction symptom; Infarct symptoms of subthalamic nucleus	丘脑底核梗死症状；丘脑底部梗死症状；丘脑底核梗塞症状；丘脑底部梗塞症状
Subtypes of Ischemic Stroke Classification System; subgroup of ischemic stroke classification system; SPARKLE	缺血性卒中分型系统亚型
Sugar-sweetened beverage; Sugar sweetened beverages; Sugar-sweetened beverages; Sugar sweetened beverage; Sugar added beverage; SSB	含糖饮料；糖饮料
Superior cerebellar artery; superior cerebellar artery; Superior cerebellar arteries; SCAs; SCA	小脑上动脉
Superior cerebellar artery embolism; Superior cerebellar artery thromboembolism; arteria cerebelli superior embolism; superior artery of cerebellum embolism	小脑上动脉栓塞；小脑上动脉血栓栓塞
Superior cerebellar artery infarction symptom; SCA infarction symptom	小脑上动脉梗死症状；小脑上动脉梗塞症状
Superoxide dismutases	超氧化物歧化酶
Superoxide radicals; Superoxides; Superoxide; O2-; O2	超氧化物；超氧阴离子

英文术语	中文术语
Susac syndrome	Susac综合征；视网膜耳蜗脑血管病变
Swallowing ability test under TV perspective	电视透视下吞咽能力检查；电视视角下的吞咽能力测试
swallowing evaluation	吞咽功能评价；吞咽功能评估
swallowing examination	吞咽检查；吞咽造影检查
swallowing rehabilitation; swallowing rehabilitation training; deglutition rehabilitation training; rehabilitation training; swallow training	吞咽康复训练；吞咽康复；吞咽障碍康复
Syncope; syncope; fainting; Faint; Blackout; Syncope attack; Fainting; Syncope (disorder)	晕厥；昏厥；厥证；晕阙；晕厥发作
Syphilitic cerebral arteritis; syphilitic cerebral arteritis; Syphilitic cerebral arteritis (disorder)	梅毒性脑动脉炎；梅毒性大脑动脉炎
Systemic hypotension; hypotension; low blood pressure; systemic hypotension; general hypotension; general low blood pressure; Systemic low blood pressure	系统性低血压；全身性低血压；低血压
Systemic lupus erythematosus arthritis; systemic lupus erythematosus arthritis; systematic lupus erythematosus arthritis; systemic lupus erythematosis arthritis; Systemic lupus erythematosus arthritis (disorder)	系统性红斑狼疮性关节炎
Systemic lupus erythmatosus; Systemic lupus erythematosus; systemic lupus erythematosus; SYSTEMIC LUPUS ERYTHEMATOSUS; SLE - Systemic lupus erythematosus; Systemic lupus erythematosus (disorder); SLE	系统性红斑狼疮；全身性红斑狼疮
Systemic vasculitis; systemic vasculitis; Systemic vasculitis (disorder); systemic vasculitides	系统性血管炎；系统性脉管炎
T lymphocytes	T淋巴细胞；T胸腺依赖性淋巴细胞；淋巴细胞；T细胞亚群；t细胞的；t淋巴；T细胞
T1-weighted images; T1 weighted images	T1加权图像
T2-weighted images; T2 weighted images	T2加权图像
Takayasu arteritis; takayasu disease	多发性大动脉炎；无脉症
Tardive dyskinesia; Drug-induced tardive dyskinesia; TD - Tardive dyskinesia; Tardive dyskinesia (disorder)	迟发性运动障碍；迟发性多动症；持续性运动障碍

续　表

英文术语	中文术语
Task-oriented therapy; Task directed therapy	任务导向治疗；任务导向疗法
Tau protein; TP	Tau蛋白
Tea intake; consumption of tea	茶摄入量；茶摄入
Tecarfarin	特卡法林
Telemedicine; remote medical; distance medical; telemedicine technology; telehealth; remote medical care	远程医疗；远程医学；远程诊疗；移动医疗；电视医学；远距会诊；远距医学；远程医疗系统
telemetry technology; Telemetry; remote sensing technology; Remote Test Technology	遥测技术；遥测
Temperature control; temperature modulated; thermal tuning; adjustment and control of temperature; thermo-regulation; temperature management	温度控制；温控；恒温控制；控温；温度调控
Temporal arteritis; temporal arteritides; cranial arteritides; Cranial arteritis; temporal arteritis; Temporal Arteritis; Temporal giant cell arteritis; TA - Temporal arteritis; Temporal arteritis (disorder)	颞动脉炎；巨细胞性颞动脉炎；颞巨细胞性动脉炎
Temporal brain region	颞脑区
Temporoparietal brain region	颞顶脑区
Temporospatial disorientation; Obstacles to spatio-temporal orientation	时空定向障碍；颞空间定向障碍
Tenecteplase	替奈普酶；替奈替普酶
Tension-type headache; Tensiontype headache; Tension headache; Tension-type headache (disorder)	紧张性头痛；紧张型头痛；肌肉收缩性头痛；肌收缩性头痛；紧缩型头痛
tertiary rehabilitation; third rehabilitative; three-level rehabilitation; three-echelon rehabilitation; three stage rehabilitation; standardized tertiary rehabilitation; three-stage rehabilitation treatment	三级康复
tertiary rehabilitation training; three-level rehabilitation training; three stage rehabilitation training	三级康复训练
Tetracycline antibiotics; tetracyclines; tetracycline; tetracycline antibiotic; tetracyclines antibiotics	四环素类抗生素；四环素菌素；四环素抗生素；四环素抗菌素
Tetraparesis; quadriparesis; Quadriparesis (disorder); Quadriparesis	四肢轻瘫
Tetraplegia; quadriplegia; tetraplegia; Paralysis of all four limbs; Quadriplegia; Quadriplegia (disorder)	四肢瘫；四肢瘫痪；四肢全瘫

英文术语	中文术语
Thalamic aphasia; thalamic aphasia, TA	丘脑性失语；丘脑失语
Thalamic dementia; Loss of psychic self activation associated with amnesia	丘脑性痴呆
Thalamic infarction syndrome; syndromes of thalamic infarction; syndrome of thalamic infarction; Thalamic infarction syndromes; Thalamic infarction symptom	丘脑梗死综合征
Thalamic pain syndrom; Dejerine Roussy syndrome	丘脑痛综合征
Thalamogeniculate artery infarction symptom; Inferolateral artery infarction symptom	丘脑膝状体动脉梗死症状；丘脑膝状体动脉梗塞症状
Thalamus; thalamus	丘脑
THAM; aminomethane; tromethamine; tris -aminomethane; tris hydroxyl methyl aminomethane	三羟甲基氨基甲烷
The Line Cancellation test; Line deletion test	线路删除测试；线路取消试验
The past functional state; The past functional condition; The past function condition; The past function states; The past functional conditions; The past function state	过去的功能状态；过去的机能状态
There was no chest pain in the first 24 hour	前 24 h 无胸痛
Thermanalgesia of the limbs and trunk; Thermal pain disorder of limbs and trunk	四肢和躯干的热性痛觉缺失；四肢和躯干的热痛觉缺失；四肢和躯干的热痛觉障碍
Thermoanesthesia; Thermal anesthesia; Thermal anaesthesia; Thermal anesthesia (finding); thermoanalgesia; thermanesthesia; thermanalgesia	温度觉缺失；温度感觉缺失；温度觉丧失
Thiazide diuretics; thiazine diuretics	噻嗪类利尿药；噻嗪类利尿剂；噻嗪利尿药
Thiazolidinedione; glitazones	噻唑烷二酮；噻唑二酮；-2,4-噻唑二酮；5-噻唑-2,4-二酮；2,4-噻唑烷二酮；噻唑烷二酮类；噻唑烷二酮类药物
Thiobarbituric acid reactive substances; TBARs	硫代巴比妥酸反应物质
Thiopental	戊硫代巴比妥；硫贲妥钠
Thrombectomy	动脉取栓术；血栓清除术；血栓摘除术；手术取栓；血栓消融术；血栓切除术

续　表

英文术语	中文术语
Thrombin activable fibrinolysis inhibitor; Thrombin-activable fibrinolysis inhibitor; plasma carboxypeptidase B; carboxypeptidase B2; TAFI	凝血酶活性纤溶抑制剂
Thrombin anti thrombin complexes; Thrombin-anti-thrombin complexes; Thrombin-antithrombin complexes	凝血酶抗凝血酶复合物
thromboembolism; embolization; embolism; Embolism (disorder); Embolism; Embolic occlusion	血栓栓塞；栓塞；栓塞性事件；血液栓塞；血管栓塞
Thrombolysis; Thrombolytic therapy; Fibrinolytic therapy; Thrombolytic drugs; Thrombolytic drug	溶栓治疗；溶栓疗法；单纯静脉溶栓；血栓溶解治疗
Thrombolysis in cerebral infarction; TICI	脑梗死时溶栓；脑梗死的溶栓治疗
Thrombomodulin; TM	血栓调节蛋白
Thrombophilia; thrombophilia; hypercoagulability; hypercoagulabale state; Hypercoagulability state (finding); Hypercoagulable state; Hypercoagulability state; Blood cloting disorder; Hypercoagulable states; prothrombotic state; Hypercoagulability; Thrombophilia (disorder)	易栓症；血栓形成倾向；高凝状态；高凝性；(血液)易凝状态；高凝固性；血栓倾向
Thromboplastin; Coagulation factor Ⅲ; Platelet tissue factor; Tissue factor; Factor Ⅲ; Factor 3; CD142; TF; thromboplastin	促凝血酶原激酶
Thrombosis; Thrombosis (disorder); thrombosis; Local occlusion	血栓形成；血栓症；易栓症
thrombospondin 1; THBS1; TSP1	血小板吸附蛋白1
Thromboxane; vasoconstrictor prostanoids; thromboxanes; thrombomodulin; thrombosis	血栓素；血栓烷；凝血烷；血栓脂质；凝血恶烷胺；凝血氧烷
Thromboxane A2; thromboxanes A2; thrombomodulin A2; thrombosis A2	血栓素A2；血栓烷A2；凝血烷A2；血栓脂质A2；凝血恶烷胺A2；凝血氧烷A2
Thunderclap headache; Thunderclap headache (disorder)	霹雳样头痛；霹雳性头痛；雷击头痛
Ticlopidine; thiamethoxam chlorine pyridine	噻氯匹定；氯苄噻啶；噻氯吡啶；噻氯匹啶[基]
Tinet balance test	Tinet平衡量表
Tinnitus; tinnitus; Ringing in ears; Noise in ears; Tinnitus (finding); Subjective tinnitus; Tinnitus aurium; Subjective tinnitus (finding)	耳鸣；耳鸣待查；耳鸣病；主觉性耳鸣；主观(性)耳鸣；主观性耳鸣
Tissue destruction markers of stroke; Tissue destruction marker of stroke	脑卒中的组织破坏标志物

英文术语	中文术语
Tissue inhibitors of metalloproteinase 1; Tissue inhibitors of metalloproteinase-1; TIMP-1; TIMP 1; TIMP1	基质金属蛋白酶抑制剂1
Tissue inhibitors of metalloproteinase 2; Tissue inhibitors of metalloproteinase-2; TIMP 2; TIMP-2; TIMP2	基质金属蛋白酶抑制剂2
Tissue inhibitors of metalloproteinases; Metalloproteinases Tissue Inhibitor; TIMP Proteins; TIMPs	基质金属蛋白酶抑制剂
Titubation; Staggering gait; Reeling gait; Staggering gait (finding)	蹒跚；蹒跚步态；步态蹒跚
Todds paralysis; Todd's paralysis; Todd's paresis; Todd paresis; Todd's paralysis; Todd's paresis (finding)	Todd麻痹；Todd麻痹；Todds瘫痪
TOF MRA; Time of flight MRA	时间飞跃法MRA；飞逝效应MRA
Toll like receptor 2; TLR2	Toll样受体2；组织细胞toll样受体2
Toll like receptor 4; TLR4	Toll样受体4；组织细胞toll样受体4
Toll like receptors; toll-like receptor	Toll样受体；组织细胞toll样受体
Toll-like receptor signaling pathway; TLR signaling pathway	Toll样受体信号通路；TLR信号通路；Toll样受体信号传导通路；Toll样受体信号转导通路
tone assessment scale; TAS	肌张力评测量表
Tongue training; lingual training; human tongue training; oral tongue training; The tongue training; palate training; linguae training; tongue squamous training	舌肌训练；舌训练
Toronto Stroke Scale	多伦多中风量表
Torsion dystonia; torsion dysmyotonia; Torsion dystonia (disorder)	扭转性肌张力障碍；扭转性张力障碍
Torticollis; Congenital torticollis; congenital torticollis; torticollis; Torticollis (disorder); torticolis; wry neck; Congenital sternomastoid torticollis; Congenital wryneck; Congenital wry neck; Congenital torticollis (disorder); Wry neck/torticollis; Wry neck/torticollis (disorder)	痉挛性斜颈；先天性斜颈；斜颈；先天性胸骨乳突肌性斜颈；先天性肌性斜颈；肌源性斜颈
Total cholesterol; Serum total cholesterol measurement; Serum total cholesterol; Serum cholesterol; Cholesterol; cholesterol	总胆固醇；降胆固醇；血脂；胆固醇含量；胆固醇
Total polyamine oxidase	总聚胺氧化酶
touch; tactile sensation; sensation; tactile; tactile sense; sense of touch	触觉；触；触摸；触感

续　表

英文术语	中文术语
Traditional Physiotherapeutic Approaches; Traditional therapy; Traditional physicotherapy; conventional physical therapy; conventional therapy; conventional physicotherapy; Traditional physical therapy	传统理疗；传统物理治疗方法
Trail Making Tests (A and B)	试运行测试（A 和 B）
Trans fat intake; trans fatty acids; Trans fat diet; Consumption of industrially produced trans fatty acids; Trans fatty acids intake; Trans fat diet intake; Trans fat food intake	反式脂肪摄入；反式脂肪摄取
transcortical aphasia	经皮质性失语；跨皮质性失语；皮质间性失语
Transcortical motor aphasia; Transcortical motor dysphasia; Transcortical motor dysphasia (disorder)	经皮质运动性失语；皮质运动性失语；皮质间运动性失语症；经皮质运动性失语症
Transcortical sensory aphasia; Transcortical sensory dysphasia; Transcortical sensory dysphasia (disorder)	经皮质感觉性失语；经皮质感觉性失语症
transcranial direct current stimulation; tDCS	经颅直流电刺激
Transcranial Doppler; TCD; doppler; transcranial doppler sonography; transcranial doppler imaging; Skull Dopplar	经颅多普勒；经颅多普勒超声；透颅多普勒；经颅超声多普勒；经颅多谱勒超声
Transcriptomics biomarkers of stroke; Gene Expressed in Blood following cerebral ischemia	脑卒中的转录组学生物标志物
Transcutaneous Electrical Nerve Stimulation; transcutaneous electric nerve stimulation	经皮电神经刺激；经皮电刺激；跨皮电刺激；体外电脉冲刺激；经皮神经电刺激；透皮神经电刺激；经皮穴位神经电刺激；透皮神经电刺激治疗
Transforming growth factor beta; TGFbeta; TGF-b; TGF-β	转化生长因子 -β
Transient ischemic attack; Transient ischaemic attack; transient ischemic attack; Impending cerebral ischemia; Minor stroke; TIAs; TIA; Transient cerebral ischemia; Transient ischemic attacks; Minor ischemic stroke; Impending cerebral ischaemia; Impending cerebral ischemia (disorder); Transient cerebral ischaemia; Intermittent cerebral ischemia; Intermittent cerebral ischaemia; Temporary cerebral vascular dysfunction; TIA - Transient ischaemic attack; Transient ischemic attack (disorder)	短暂性脑缺血发作；短暂性大脑缺血；短暂性缺血发作；短暂脑缺血；短暂性大脑缺血性发作；短暂脑缺血发作；暂时性局部缺血发作；小中风；暂时性脑局部缺血；短暂性脑缺血；暂时性脑缺血

英文术语	中文术语
Transthyretin; Prealbumin; TTR	甲状腺素运载蛋白
Trauma; trauma; Wound; Wound (disorder); Head trauma; Traumatic injury; Traumatic injury (disorder)	创伤；创伤病；外伤性损伤；创伤性损伤
Treatment; Therapeutics; Treatments; Therapies; Therapy; treatment	治疗；疗法；治疗方法
Treatment of atherosclerotic cerebrovascular disease	动脉粥样硬化性脑血管病的治疗
Treatment of pain and anxiety	治疗疼痛和焦虑；疼痛和焦虑的治疗
treatment scheme; treatment plan; treatment planning; treatment planning system; radiotherapy plan; therapy planning	治疗方案；治疗计划；处治方案
Tremor; tremor; Fremitus; Trembling; Shaking; Fremitus (finding); Thrill; Thrill (finding); Shakes; The shakes; Tremor (finding)	震颤；颤振病
Tremor by anatomical site	按解剖部位分类的震颤
Trial of ORG 10172 in acute stroke treatment; TOAST	TOAST 分型；ORG 10172 在急性脑卒中治疗中的试验
Triflusal	三氟柳；对三氟甲基乙酰水杨酸；三氟醋柳酸
Triglycerides; triacylglycerol; triglycercide; triglyceride; Triglyceride	甘油三酯；三酰甘油
Triglycerides measurement; Determination of triglyceride	甘油三酯测量；甘油三酯测定
Tritanomaly; tritanomalia; Tritan defect; Tritan defect (disorder)	蓝色弱；蓝色盲
Truncal ataxia; Truncal ataxia (finding)	躯干性共济失调；躯干共济失调
Truncal titubation	躯干蹒跚；Truncal 蹒跚步态
Truncular ataxia; Trunk ataxia	闭合性共济失调
trunk control test; TCT	躯干控制测验；躯干控制试验
Tuberothalamic artery infarction symptom; Anterior thalamic infarction symptom; Polar artery infarction symptom	丘脑结节动脉梗死症状；丘脑结节动脉梗塞症状
Tumor necrosis factor alpha; tumor necrosis factor a; TNF-alpha; cachectin; TNF alpha; cachexin; TNF a; TNFa	肿瘤坏死因子 a；恶病质素
Tumor necrosis factor beta; Tumor Necrosis Factor-beta; alpha Lymphotoxin; Lymphotoxin-alpha; Lymphotoxin alpha; Lymphotoxin; TNF-beta; TNF beta; TNF-b; TNF b	肿瘤坏死因子 β；α 淋巴毒素
Turn over regularly; Turn over timed; Turn over timing	定时翻身；定期翻身；规律翻身

续 表

英文术语	中文术语
Turnip; Turnips	芜菁；萝卜
Type 2 Diabetes mellitus; Type 2 DM; T2DM	2型糖尿病
Type Ⅰ Hyperlipoproteinemia; C-Ⅱ Anapolipoproteinemias; Familial LPL Deficiencies; C-Ⅱ Anapolipoproteinemia; Familial Chylomicronemia; Familial LPL Deficiency; Burger-Grutz Syndromes; Burger Grutz Syndrome; Lipase D Deficiencies; Lipase D Deficiency; LIPD Deficiency; Hyperlipoproteinemia Type I; Familial Fat Induced Hypertriglyceridemia; Familial Lipoprotein Lipase Deficiency; Familial Hyperlipoproteinemia Type 1; Lipoprotein Lipase Deficiencies; Apolipoprotein C Ⅱ Deficiency; Familial Hyperchylomicronemias; Familial Hyperchylomicronemia; Lipoprotein Lipase Deficiency; Type I Hyperlipoproteinemias	高脂蛋白血症Ⅰ型；脂蛋白脂酶缺乏；家族性高乳糜微粒血症；家族性脂蛋白脂酶缺乏症；载脂蛋白CⅡ缺乏；伯格-格鲁茨综合征
Type Ⅱ Hyperlipoproteinemia; LDL Receptor Disorder; Hyperlipoproteinemia Type Ⅱ; Familial Hypercholesterolemic Xanthomatoses; Familial Hypercholesterolemic Xanthomatosis; Familial Combined Hyperlipoproteinemias; Autosomal Dominant Hypercholesterolemia; Familial Combined Hyperlipoproteinemia; Hyper Low Density Lipoproteinemia; Essential Hypercholesterolemias; Essential Hypercholesterolemia; Familial Hypercholesterolemias; Familial Hypercholesterolemia; Hyperlipoproteinemia Type 2; Hyper beta Lipoproteinemia; Hyperbetalipoproteinemias; Hyperbetalipoproteinemia; LDL Receptor Disorders; high β lipoprotein; Hyperbetalipoproteinaemia; Hyperbetalipoproteinemia (disorder)	高脂蛋白血症Ⅱ型；高β-脂蛋白血症；β-脂蛋白过高；β脂蛋白血过高

英文术语	中文术语
Type Ⅲ Hyperlipoproteinemia; Hyperlipoproteinemia Type Ⅲ; Familial Hypercholesterolemia with Hyperlipemia; Broad-beta Hyperlipoproteinemia; Familial Dysbetalipoproteinemia; Type Ⅲ Hyperlipoproteinemias; Dysbetalipoproteinemia; Broad Beta Disease; Familial type 3 hyperlipoproteinemia; Familial type 3 hyperlipoproteinaemia; Remnant hyperlipoproteinemia; Familial dysbetalipoproteinaemia; Familial type Ⅲ hyperlipoproteinaemia; Fredrickson type Ⅲ hyperlipoproteinaemia; Fredrickson type Ⅲ hyperlipoproteinemia; Remnant hyperlipidaemia; Remnant hyperlipidemia; Remnant hyperlipoproteinaemia; Familial hyperbetalipoproteinaemia and hyperprebetalipoproteinaemia; Familial hyperbetalipoproteinemia and hyperprebetalipoproteinemia; Familial hypercholesterolaemia with hyperlipaemia; Familial hypercholesterolemia with hyperlipemia; Familial type 3 hyperlipoproteinemia (disorder)	高脂蛋白血症Ⅲ型；家族性 3 型高脂蛋白血症；残粒移去障碍病；Ⅲ型高脂蛋白血症；残粒性血脂蛋白过多症；家族性3型高脂蛋白血症；家族性3型血脂蛋白过多症；家族性血β脂蛋白异常症；血β脂蛋白异常；宽β脂蛋白病；家族性异常β脂蛋白血症；宽β病；β-脂蛋白不良血症；宽β疾病；β脂蛋白不良血症；残粒高脂血症；家族性β-脂蛋白不良血症；血β脂蛋白异常
Type Ⅳ Hyperlipoproteinemia; Hyperlipoproteinemia Type Ⅳ; Familial Type Ⅳ Hyperlipoproteinemia; Familial Hyperlipoproteinemia Type 4; Carbohydrate Inducible Hyperlipemias; Carbohydrate Inducible Hyperlipemia; Hyper prebeta lipoproteinemia; Familial Hypertriglyceridemia; Type Ⅳ Hyperlipoproteinemias; Hyperprebetalipoproteinemia	高脂蛋白血症Ⅳ型；碳水化合物诱导的高脂血症；家族性Ⅳ型高脂蛋白血症
Type of free radicals; Types of free radical; category of free radicals; Types of radicals; category of radicals	自由基的类型
Type V Hyperlipoproteinemia; Hyperlipoproteinemia Type V; Hyperchylomicronemia Late Onsets; Hyperchylomicronemia Late Onset; Late-Onset Hyperchylomicronemia; Type V Hyperlipoproteinemias; Hyperlipoproteinemia Type 5; Type V Hyperlipidemias; Type V Hyperlipidemia; Mixed Hyperlipemias; Mixed Hyperlipemia	高脂蛋白血症Ⅴ型；晚发性高乳糜微粒血症；混合型高脂血症
Types of rehabilitation; species of rehabilitation; kinds of rehabilitation; category of rehabilitation	康复类型；康复种类
Tyrosine; Tyr; Increase of tyrosine; tyrosine	酪氨酸；酪氨酸增加；3-对羟苯基丙氨酸
Ubiquitin fusion degradation protein; UB fusion protein 1; UFD1L; UFDP	泛素融合降解蛋白
UGT1A1; UDP glucuronosyltransferase family 1 member A1	尿苷磷酸葡萄糖醛酸转移酶1A1

续　表

英文术语	中文术语
UGT1A1*28 polymorphism；UGT1A1-28 polymorphism；UGT1A1*28 polymorphism (disorder)	UGT1A1*28基因多态性
Ultrasound methods；Ultrasound technique；Ultrasound	超声检查；超声方法；超声；超声波；超声图
Unfavorable outcome；Worse outcomes；Poor outcomes；Worse outcome	预后不佳；不良结局；转归不良；疗效差；结局不佳
Unilateral deafness；single sided deafness；single side deafness；Unilateral hearing loss	单耳聋；单侧耳聋
Unilateral ptosis；one side ptosis；single lateral ptosis；unilateral side ptosis；single-sided ptosis；mono-side ptosis	单侧上睑下垂；一侧上睑下垂
Unilateral weakness	单侧肢体无力；单边软弱；单侧软弱
Unsaturated fats；Unsaturated fatty acids	不饱和脂肪；不饱和脂肪酸
Up regulated gene after brain ischemia；specifically up-regulated after brain ischemia	脑缺血后上调基因；脑缺血后基因上调
Upbeat nystagmus；Upbeat central vestibular nystagmus；Upbeat central nystagmus；Upbeat nystagmus (disorder)；Upbeat central vestibular nystagmus (disorder)	上跳性眼震；上跳性眼球震颤；上视性眼球震颤；眼球下跃式垂直性眼震
upper extremity strength；upper limb muscle strength；upper limb's muscle strength	上肢肌力；上肢肌肉力量
Upper limb postural tremor；Postural tremor of upper limbs	上肢姿势性震颤；上肢震颤；上肢体位性震颤
Upper quadrantanopsia without cognitive impairment；Upper quadrantanopsia without cognitive disturbance；quadrantic hemianopia；Upper quadrantanopsia without cognition disorders；Upper quadrantanopsia without cognitive dysfunction	无认知障碍的上象限盲；上象限盲无认知障碍
Uric acid；Uric acid levels；Uric acid level；Serum uric acid；SUA	尿酸
Urinalysis；UA；urine analysis；urinal；urine urinalysis；urinalysis	尿常规；尿分析法；尿沉渣分析；尿生化；尿检；尿分析
Urinary tract infection；UTI；Urinary tract infectious disease；UTI - Urinary tract infection；Urinary tract infectious disease (disorder)	泌尿系感染；泌尿道感染性疾病；尿路感染；泌尿道感染；泌尿系统感染；尿道感染
Urokinase；urokinase	尿激酶

英文术语	中文术语
Vascular cell adhesion molecule 1; Vascular cell adhesion molecule-1; VCAM-1	血管细胞黏附分子1
Vascular disorder; Vascular disease; Disorder of blood vessel; Angiopathy; Vascular disease (disorder); Disorder of blood vessel (disorder)	血管性疾病；血管病症；血管病；血管病变；血管疾病
Vascular disorder due to drug abuse; Vascular diseases caused by drug abuse	药物滥用引起的血管疾病；药物滥用引起的血管紊乱
vascular endothelial growth factor A; VEGFA	血管内皮生长因子A
Vascular imaging; Cerebrovascular imaging; angiography; ct angiography; angiography imaging; blood vessel imaging; vessel imaging	血管成像；血管成像技术；CT血管成像；血管影像学；血管影像
Vascular parkinsonism; vascular Parkinsonism; vascular Parkinsinism; vascular ischemic parkinsonism; cerebral vascular disease and parkinsonism; Vascular parkinsonism (disorder)	血管性帕金森综合征；血管性帕金森综合症；血管性帕金森病；血管性帕金森症
Vasogenic edema; angio-edema; vasogenic; angioedema; angioneurotic edema	血管源性水肿；血管性水肿
Vasovagal syncope; vasovagal syncope; Neurally-mediated syncope; Vasodepressor syncope; Vasovagal attack; Gower's syndrome; Vaso vagal episode; Vasovagal syncope (disorder); Vasovagal syncope (finding)	血管迷走神经性晕厥；血管迷走性晕厥；血管减压药性晕厥；迷走血管性晕厥；血管抑制性晕厥；血管减压性晕厥；血管减压型晕厥；血管迷走神经型晕厥；血管迷走神经晕厥；血管神经性晕厥；迷走反射性晕厥；血管减压药晕厥
Vasulitis; inflammation of blood vessels; Vasculitides; Angiitis; Vasculitis; Vasculitis (disorder)	血管炎；血管炎(脉管炎)；血管炎(病)；脉管炎
Vegetable; consumption of vegetables; consumption of vegetable; dietary vegetable; Vegetables	蔬菜；菜
Venous thromboembolism; venous embolism; Venous embolism; Embolism of vein; venous thromboembolism; Thromboembolism of vein; Venous embolism (disorder); Venous thromboembolic disease; Thromboembolism of vein (disorder)	静脉栓塞；静脉血栓；静脉血栓栓塞；静脉血栓栓塞症；静脉血栓栓子疾病
Venous thrombosis; Phlebothrombosis; venous thrombosis; phlebothrombosis; Venous thrombosis (disorder)	静脉血栓形成

续　表

英文术语	中文术语
verbal; parole; discourse; spoken language; rhetoric; utterance; saying; speech	言语；讲话；言说；话语；语言
Vertebral artery; Vertebral Artery; arteria vertebralis; vertebral artery; Vertebral arteries; VAs; VA	椎动脉
Vertebral artery atherosclerosis; Vertebral atherosclerotic plaque; vertebral atherosclerosis; vertebrarterial atherosclerosis; vertebral artery	椎动脉粥样硬化；椎动脉粥样硬化斑块
Vertebral artery dissection; VAD; Dissection of vertebral artery; Dissection of vertebral artery (disorder); Vertebral artery dissection (disorder)	椎动脉夹层
Vertebral artery embolism; vertebral artery embolism; Vertebral artery embolus; Vertebral artery embolism (disorder); Vertebral artery thromboembolism	椎动脉栓塞；椎动脉血栓栓塞
Vertebral artery infarction symptom; Medullary infarct symptom; Symptoms of vertebral artery infarction	椎动脉梗死症状；椎动脉梗塞症状；髓样梗塞症状
Vertebrobasilar dolichoectasia; Basilar artery syndrome (disorder); Basilar artery syndrome; Insufficiency - basilar artery; Vertebrobasilar arterial insufficiency; Vertebrobasilar insufficiency; Dolichoectasia; VBD	椎基底动脉延长扩张症；基底动脉综合征；椎底动脉供血不足；椎基底动脉供血不足；基底动脉综合症
Vertebrobasilar infarction syndrome; syndromes of vertebrobasilar infarction; syndrome of vertebrobasilar infarction; Vertebrobasilar infarction syndromes; Vertebrobasilar infarction symptom; VB infarction symptom	椎基底动脉梗死综合征
Vertical gaze paresis; Disorders of vertical gaze	垂直注视麻痹；垂直注视障碍
Vertical nystagmus; vertical nystagmus; Vertical nystagmus (disorder)	垂直性眼震；垂直眼球震颤；垂直性眼球震颤；垂直眼震
Vertigo; Dizziness (finding); dizziness; Dizziness; vertigo; Rotary vertigo; Rotatory vertigo	眩晕；头昏；头晕；眩晕症
Very low density lipoprotein Cholesterol; Prebetalipoprotein Cholesterol; VLDL Cholesterol; VLDL	极低密度脂蛋白胆固醇
Vestibular nystagmus; Nystagmus associated with disorder of the vestibular system; Nystagmus associated with disorders of the vestibular system; Nystagmus associated with disorder of the vestibular system (disorder)	前庭性眼震；前庭性眼球震颤；前庭性眼振；前庭眼球震颤；与前庭系统疾病有关的眼球震颤

续 表

英文术语	中文术语
Virtual Reality; virtual reality; VR; virtual reality modeling; visual reality; virtual realization; virtue reality; virtual reality technology	虚拟现实；虚拟现实技术；虚拟仿真；虚拟环境
Visinin like protein 1; Visinin-like protein-1; VLP-1	视锥蛋白样蛋白 -1
vision; visual; visual sense; visional; perception; perception, visual ; visual function; sense of sight	视觉；视觉功能；视力功能
Visual agnosia; Visuoperceptual agnosia; Visual agnosia (disorder)	视觉失认；视觉失认症；视失知症；视觉不识症
Visual Attention Training; vision Attention Training	视觉注意力训练；视觉关注训练
visual exploration therapy; Visual scanning training	视觉探索疗法；视觉扫描训练
Visual Field; visual fields; view; perspective; field of vision; field of view; range of vision; visual field	视野；视域；视界
Visual field defect; vision field defect; defect of visual field; visual field defect; VFD - Visual field defect; Visual field defect (finding)	视野缺损；视野缺失；视野缺陷；视野损害；视觉缺陷
Visual hallucinations; Visual illusions; visual hallucination; Visual Hallucinations; Visual hallucination; Seeing things; Visual hallucinations (finding)	视幻觉；幻视
Visual impairment; visual disturbance; Vision disorder; Visual impairments; visual disorder; Visual impairment (disorder); Disorder of vision (disorder); Impaired vision; Visual disturbance (disorder); Disorder of vision; Visual disturbance	视觉障碍；视力受损；视力障碍
Vital signs; Signs of life; Vital sign	生命征象；生命指征；生命指标；生命体征
vital signs were stable for 24 hour	生命体征稳定达 24 h
Vitamin A intake; Vitamin A supplements	维生素 A 摄入量
Vitamin B intake; Vitamin B_{12} intake; Vitamin B_1 intake; Vitamin B_6 intake; B vitamins intake; Vitamin B_2 intake	维生素 B 摄入量
Vitamin D intake	维生素 D 摄入量
Vitamin E intake; Vitamin E supplements	维生素 E 摄入量
Vitamin intake; Antioxidant vitamins; Multivitamin pill; Antioxidant pill	维生素摄入
Vivid hallucinations; vivid illusion	幻觉生动；强烈的幻觉；逼真的幻觉
Voice tremor; Vocal tremor; Voice tremor (finding)	声音震颤；声音颤抖；声带震颤

续　表

英文术语	中文术语
Vomiting; vomit; vomiting; Vomit; vomition; Emesis; Finding of vomiting; Observation of vomiting; Finding of vomiting (finding); Vomiting (disorder)	呕吐；呕吐症状
von Willebrand factor; von Willebrand Protein; Factor VIII vWF; vWF	血管性假血友病因子；冯.维勒布兰德因子
Walking; walk; on foot; perambulation; perambulate; hike; step; gait; walking	步行；行走；步行的；竞走；慢步；走步；走
walking ability; stepping ability; ambulation ability; walk ability; walking abilities; walking capability	行走能力；步行能力；步行功能；行路能力
Wallenberg syndrome; Dorsolateral medullary infarction symptom; Laterodorsal medullary infarction symptom; LMI	延髓背外侧综合征
Warfarin; Panwarfin; Coumadin; Sofarin	华法林；丙酮苄羟香豆素；苄酮香豆素钠 华法林；苄丙酮香豆素 华法林；华法灵
Water swallow Test	洼田饮水测试；Watian饮水测试
Water-Based Exercises; aquatic sports; water sport; nautics; aquatic; water movement; aquatics sports; aquatics; Water sports	水上锻炼；水上活动；水上运动
Watershed infarction syndrome; syndromes of watershed infarction; syndrome of watershed infarction; Watershed infarction syndromes; borderzone infarction symptom; Watershed infarction symptom	分水岭梗死综合征
Wavelete CTA	小波CTA
Weakness of the proximal limbs; proximal limb weakness; weakness of proximal extremities; weakness of proximal limbs	近端肢体无力；四肢近端无力；近端四肢无力
Weber syndrome; weber syndrome; Weber Syndrome	韦伯氏综合征(大脑脚综合征)；韦伯综合征；大脑脚综合征；韦伯(氏)综合征；韦伯（氏）综合征；动眼神经交叉瘫
Wechsler memory scale; WMS	韦氏记忆量表
Wegener granulomatosis; Wegener's granulomatosis; Granulomatosis with polyangiitis; Wegener's granulomatosis (disorder); Granulomatosis with polyangiitis (disorder)	韦格纳肉芽肿病；韦格纳肉芽肿；肉芽肿性多血管炎；韦氏肉芽肿病；韦格内肉芽肿；韦格内氏肉芽肿；Wegener肉芽肿；肉芽肿性血管炎；Wegener肉芽肿病

续　表

英文术语	中文术语
Weight loss; Healthy body weight; Healthy weight; weight loss	减重；体重减轻；减肥；体重下降
Wernicke's aphasia; Wernicke-type aphasia; Jargon dysphasia; Receptive dysphasia; Receptive aphasia; Posterior dysphasia; Wernicke's dysphasia; Wernicke's aphasia; Receptive dysphasia (disorder)	Wernicke失语；接受型语言障碍；韦尼克失语
Western Aphasia Battery; WAB-R; WAB	西方失语症成套测验
Wheelchairs; invalid chair; wheelchair	轮椅；轮椅车
White blood cell; white blood cell; leukocyte; WBC	白细胞；白血球
Whole body coordination training; Whole-body coordination training	全身协调性训练；全身协调训练；整体协调训练
Willingness to participate in rehabilitation treatment; intention to participate in rehabilitation treatment; intention to attendance rehabilitation treatment; Willingness to attendance rehabilitation treatment	参加康复治疗的意愿；愿意参与康复治疗
Wolf Motor Function Test; WMFT	Wolf运动功能测试
World federation of neurological surgeons scale; WFNS scale	世界神经外科医生联合会量表
Writer's cramp; writer's cramp; writing spasm; Graphospasm; Writers' cramp; Scriveners' palsy; Writers' paralysis; Writers' spasm	书写痉挛；书写痉挛症；器质性书写痉挛；书写麻痹；书写痉挛(器质性)；书写性痉挛症；书写性麻痹

附录B

动脉粥样硬化性脑血管病术语定义

英文术语（中文术语）	定义（英文和/或中文）
Abasia(行走不稳)	A severe form of gait ataxia such that an affected person cannot walk at all [2]
Abasia(行走不稳)	明显的步态共济失调，导致受累者无法行走[2]
abciximab(阿昔单抗)	Abciximab (ReoPro) is the Fab fragment of a chimeric human/mouse monoclonal antibody directed against the platelet glycoprotein Ⅱb/Ⅲa (GP Ⅱb/Ⅲa) receptor, the final mediator of aggregation. Abciximab appears to be safe when administered up to 24 hours after stroke onset, and it might improve functional outcome[1]
Abnormal Amsler grid test(阿姆斯勒方格表检查异常)	Abnormal Amsler grid test [2]
Abnormal Amsler grid test(阿姆斯勒方格表检查异常)	阿姆斯勒方格表检查异常[2]
Abnormal automated kinetic perimetry test(自动动态视野检查异常)	Abnormal automated kinetic perimetry test [2]
Abnormal automated kinetic perimetry test(自动动态视野检查异常)	自动动态视野检查异常[2]
Abnormal confrontational visual field test(异常对抗视野测试)	Abnormal confrontational visual field test [2]
Abnormal confrontational visual field test(异常对抗视野测试)	面对面视野检查异常[2]
Abnormal Estermann grid perimetry test(Estermann 网格视野检查异常)	Abnormal Estermann grid perimetry test [2]

［1］ HABIBI-KOOLAEE M, SHAHMORADI L, NIAKAN KALHORI S R, et al. STO: stroke ontology for accelerating translational stroke research［J］. Neurol Ther, 2021, 10(1): 321-333.
［2］ 中国人类表型本体/Human Phenotype Ontology China(HPCH)［EB/OL］.（2019-11-22）. http://medportal.bmicc.cn/ontologies/HPCH.
［3］ 医学名词审定委员会, 物理医学与康复名词审定分委员会. 物理医学与康复名词［M］. 北京 : 科学出版社, 2014.

英文术语（中文术语）	定义（英文和/或中文）
Abnormal Estermann grid perimetry test(Estermann 网格视野检查异常)	Estermann 网格视野检查异常[2]
Abnormal Humphrey SITA 10-2 perimetry test(Humphrey SITA 10-2 视野检查异常)	Abnormal Humphrey SITA 10-2 perimetry test[2]
Abnormal Humphrey SITA 10-2 perimetry test(Humphrey SITA 10-2 视野检查异常)	Humphrey SITA 10-2 视野检查异常[2]
Abnormal Humphrey SITA 24-2 perimetry test(Humphrey SITA 24-2 视野检查异常)	Abnormal Humphrey SITA 24-2 perimetry test[2]
Abnormal Humphrey SITA 24-2 perimetry test(Humphrey SITA 24-2 视野检查异常)	Humphrey SITA 24-2 视野检查异常[2]
Abnormal Humphrey SITA 30-2 perimetry test(Humphrey SITA 30-2 视野检查异常)	Abnormal Humphrey SITA 30-2 perimetry test[2]
Abnormal Humphrey SITA 30-2 perimetry test(Humphrey SITA 30-2 视野检查异常)	Humphrey SITA 30-2 视野检查异常[2]
Abnormal kinetic perimetry test(动态视野检查异常)	Abnormal kinetic perimetry test[2]
Abnormal kinetic perimetry test(动态视野检查异常)	动态视野检查异常[2]
Abnormal manual kinetic perimetry test(手工动态视野检查异常)	Abnormal manual kinetic perimetry test[2]
Abnormal manual kinetic perimetry test(手工动态视野检查异常)	手工动态视野检查异常[2]
Abnormal static automated perimetry test(自动静态视野检查异常)	Abnormal static automated perimetry test[2]
Abnormal static automated perimetry test(自动静态视野检查异常)	自动静态视野检查异常[2]
Abnormal static perimetry test(静态视野检查异常)	Abnormal static perimetry test[2]
Abnormal static perimetry test(静态视野检查异常)	静态视野检查异常[2]
Abnormal visual field test(视野检查异常)	Abnormal visual field test[2]
Abnormal visual field test(视野检查异常)	视野检查异常[2]
Action tremor(动作性震颤)	A tremor present when the limbs are active, either when outstretched in a certain position or throughout a voluntary movement[2]

续　表

英文术语（中文术语）	定义（英文和/或中文）
Action tremor(动作性震颤)	当肢体处于活动状态，或者当肢体伸出在某个位置或在自主运动过程中出现的震颤[2]
active exercise(主动运动)	患者在无外力作用的情况下主动独立完成运动的训练方式。以增强肌力和耐力、改善关节功能、心肺功能和全身状况。可作为肌力3级患者的肌力训练[3]
Acute agitated delirium(急性躁狂性谵妄)	Acute agitated delirium is probably a result of damage to the right middle temporal gyrus and inferior parietal lobule[1]
Adjusted clinical group(调整临床组)	ACGs were originally developed to predict ambulatory care visits among patients of health maintenance organizations but have since been widely used to describe the extent of medical problems and their likely effects on health care resource use. Each ICD-9-CM code for a patient is assigned to 1 of 32 mutually exclusive adjusted diagnosis groups that groups diagnoses based on their similarity on a number of characteristics including expected persistence of the condition, likelihood of requiring hospitalization, or need for specialty referral[1]
Akathisia(静坐不能)	Akathisia per se has not been reported in association with stroke, except in one case of unilateral akathisia in a posterior thalamic infarct. Cases of agitation or agitated confusional state have also been reported in association with various locations especially subthalamic infarcts but also caudate hemorrhagic and ischemic strokes, mesencephalic and substantia nigra, thalamic, right hemispheric or multiple lacunar strokes[1]
Akinetic mutism(无动性缄默)	The term akinetic mutism was coined by Cairns to describe a patient with an epidermoid cyst of the third ventricle, who was mute and immobile, but followed with her eyes the observer as well as moving objects and who could be brought by repetitive stimulation to "whisper few onosyllables" and "slow feeble voluntary movements", in the absence of "gross alterations of sensory–motor mechanisms operating at a more peripheral level". Akinetic mutism (a.m.) represents an extreme form of abulia (abulia major) due to disruption of reticulothalamofrontal and extrathalamic reticulo-frontal afferents. Two forms of a.m. have been identified. The first variety of a.m. has been described in patients with bilateral occlusion of the anterior cerebral arteries and hemorrhages (with vasospasm) from anterior communicating aneurysms[1]

英文术语（中文术语）	定义（英文和/或中文）
Albert Test(艾伯特测试)	Albert's test is a straightforward, easily quantifiable test for the presence of neglect in stroke, and compliance is high even early in stroke. It is a useful addition to the battery of tests for the clinical assessment of perceptual disorder in stroke and its quantifiable nature is especially relevant to charting progress in the patient undergoing rehabilitation. It would be of value as a standardised test for neglect in further stroke research [1]
Alberta stroke program early CT score(艾伯塔中风计划早期CT评分)	The Alberta stroke programe early CT score (ASPECTS) 1 is a 10-point quantitative topographic CT scan score used in patients with middle cerebral artery (MCA) stroke. Segmental assessment of the MCA vascular territory is made and 1 point is deducted from the initial score of 10 for every region involved: caudate putamen internal capsule insular cortex M1: "anterior MCA cortex," corresponding to frontal operculum M2: "MCA cortex lateral to insular ribbon" corresponding to anterior temporal lobe M3: "posterior MCA cortex" corresponding to posterior temporal lobe M4: "anterior MCA territory immediately superior to M1" M5: "lateral MCA territory immediately superior to M2" M6: "posterior MCA territory immediately superior to M3" [1]
Alcohol drinking(饮酒)	Behaviors associated with the ingesting of alcoholic beverages, including social drinking [1]
Alcohol drinking(饮酒)	The guidelines for the prevention of stroke recommend the consumption of a maximum of 2 alcoholic drinks per day for men and 1 alcoholic drink per day for non-pregnant women [1]
Alexia without agraphia syndrome(失读不伴失写综合征)	When the reading deficit occurs in the absence of other reading, writing or spelling deficits, it is referred to as "pure alexia" or, as originally defined by Déjerine, "pure word blindness" [1]
alpha 2 macroglobulin(α 2巨球蛋白)	a2-macroglobulin plays a role as a carrier protein for IL-6, protecting the cytokine from degradative proteases in the plasma [1]

续　表

英文术语（中文术语）	定义（英文和/或中文）
Alpha tocopherol(维生素 E)	A natural tocopherol and one of the most potent antioxidant tocopherols. It exhibits antioxidant activity by virtue of the phenolic hydrogen on the 2H-1-benzopyran-6-ol nucleus. It has four methyl groups on the 6-chromanol nucleus. The natural d form of alpha-tocopherol is more active than its synthetic dl-alpha-tocopherol racemic mixture [1]
Altitudinal visual field defect(垂直视野缺损)	Altitudinal visual field defect [2]
Altitudinal visual field defect(垂直视野缺损)	垂直视野缺损 [2]
Amaurosis fugax(一过性黑矇)	sudden onset of a fog, haze, scum, curtain, shade, blur, cloud or mist [1]
Amphetamine(安非他明)	Amphetamine (contracted from alpha-methylphenethylamine) is a potent central nervous system (CNS) stimulant that is used in the treatment of attention deficit hyperactivity disorder (ADHD), narcolepsy, and obesity [1]
Amsterdam Nijmegen Everyday Language Test(Amsterdam Nijmegen 日常语言测试)	he ANELT is designed to assess the level of verbal communicative abilities of individuals with aphasia [1]
Amusia(失音症)	Perception of music is impaired in most patients with auditory sound agnosia, but a disproportionate difficulty in recognizing melodies is referred to as sensory (or receptive) amusia [1]
Anarthria(构音障碍)	Anarthria is due to bilateral facio-glosso-pharyngo-laryngeal paralysis, which also causes dysphagia and limits the use of facial expression in communication [1]
Ancrod(安克洛酶)	Ancrod, an enzyme derived from snake venom that degrades fibrinogen, was tested in a series of clinical studies [1]
Angioplasty(血管成形术)	Balloon angioplasty with or without stent placement represents a different approach to the recanalization of arterial occlusion. This strategy, which is similar to the approach commonly taken in patients with acute myocardial infarction, was hampered for a long time by the absence of dedicated catheters for the cerebral vasculature [1]
Anisocoria(瞳孔不等)	Anisocoria, or unequal pupil size, may represent a benign physiologic variant or a manifestation of disease. Pathologic anisocoria can reflect an abnormality of the musculature of the iris or of the sympathetic or prasympathetic innervation of the iris [1]

续　表

英文术语（中文术语）	定义（英文和/或中文）
Anomalous trichromacy(三色视觉障碍)	Individuals with anomalous trichromacy possess three types of cones, but one of the three types of cones has an abnormal spectral sensitivity compared to normal cones [2]
Anomalous trichromacy(三色视觉障碍)	三色视异常的患者具有三种类型的视锥细胞，但三种视锥细胞中的一种相对于正常视锥细胞光谱灵敏度异常 [2]
Anosodiaphoria(疾病淡漠)	Anosodiaphoria is a condition in which a person who suffers disability due to brain injury seems indifferent to the existence of their handicap. Anosodiaphoria is specifically used in association with indifference to paralysis. It is a somatosensory agnosia, or a sign of neglect syndrome [1]
Anosognosia(疾病失认症)	The term anosognosia was introduced in 1914 by Anton and Babinski to denote lack of interest and concern for deficits relative to the left hemispace. Typically a patient may deny left hemiplegia or left hemianopia. There appears to be no causal link with hemineglect, since anosognosia was reported in cases without hemineglect [1]
Anterior cerebral artery infarction syndrome (大脑前动脉梗死综合征)	The ACA is subdivided into the A1 segment (before the anterior communicating artery (ACoA), followed by the A2 segment (after the ACoA), then A3 segments. The A1 segment has deep perforating arteries, named the medial lenticulostriate arteries, and gives rise to the recurrent artery of Heubner (raH), which supplies the caudate head, the genu and anterior arm of the internal capsule and the supero-anterior putamen. Both the lenticulostriate arteries and the raH are particularly vulnerable during aneurysm surgery of the ACoA [1]
Anterior choroidal artery infarction syndrome (脉络膜前动脉梗死综合征)	Lacunar syndrome within AChA territory causes most frequently pure motor or sensorimotor hemiparesis. A rarer but typical presentation of AChA infarcts is the triad of contralateral severe hemiparesis, hemihypesthesia and upper quadrantanopsia [1]
Anterior inferior cerebellar artery infarction symptom(小脑前下动脉梗死症状)	The AICA vascularizes the dorsolateral inferior pons, the antero-inferior cerebellum, the cochlea, the labyrinth, and the VIIIth cranial nerve [1]
Anterograde amnesia(顺行性遗忘)	Anterograde amnesia is an inability to recall or recognize events, facts, or concepts to which one was exposed following the onset of illness [1]

135

续　表

英文术语（中文术语）	定义（英文和/或中文）
anticoagulants(抗凝剂)	Anticoagulant therapy for acute stroke may only be considered after a brain imaging study has excluded hemorrhage and estimated the size of the infarct. Early anticoagulation should be avoided when potential contraindications to anticoagulation are present, such as a large infarction (based upon clinical syndrome or brain imaging findings), uncontrolled hypertension, or other bleeding conditions[1]
Antioxidants(抗氧化剂)	Naturally occurring or synthetic substances that inhibit or retard oxidation reactions. They counteract the damaging effects of oxidation in animal tissues[1]
Antiphospholipid syndrome(抗磷脂抗体综合征)	Antiphospholipid syndrome (APS) is defined by the development of thrombosis and/or adverse obstetric events in the presence of antiphospholipid antibodies (aPL)[1]
Apathy(淡漠)	Apathy is a frequent neuropsychiatric complication of stroke that, although often associated with depression and cognitive impairment, may occur independently of both. Its presence has been consistently associated with greater functional decline[1]
Aphasic Depression Rating Scale(失语抑郁量表)	ADRS is a valid, reliable, sensitive, and specific tool for the evaluation of depression in aphasic patients during the stroke subacute phase[1]
Apixaban(阿哌沙班)	Apixaban is a small molecule that acts as a selective inhibitor of factor Xa, which is a key coagulation factor located at the junction of the extrinsic and intrinsic pathways of the coagulation cascade[1]
APOE(载脂蛋白E)	only the APOE gene has been identified as a robust genetic risk factor for intracerebral hemorrhage. APOE is considered a strong risk factor for cerebral amyloid angiopathy and it is for a large part via this underlying etiology that APOE relates with intracerebral hemorrhage. However, APOE has also been shown to affect blood vessels via other mechanisms[1]

续　表

英文术语（中文术语）	定义（英文和/或中文）
Apolipoprotein C1(载脂蛋白C1)	A 6.6-kDa protein component of VERY-LOW-DENSITY LIPOPROTEINS; INTERMEDIATE-DENSITY LIPOPROTEINS; and HIGH-DENSITY LIPOPROTEINS. Apo C-I displaces APO E from lipoproteins, modulate their binding to receptors (RECEPTORS, LDL), and thereby decrease their clearance from plasma. Elevated Apo C-I levels are associated with HYPERLIPOPROTEINEMIA and ATHEROSCLEROSIS[1]
Apolipoprotein C3(载脂蛋白C3)	Apolipoprotein C-III (99 aa, ~11 kDa) is encoded by the human APOC3 gene. This protein is involved in the modulation of cellular uptake and metabolism of very low density lipoproteins and chylomicrons[1]
Apoptosis(细胞凋亡)	Apoptosis is an energy-consuming process, so reperfusion could potentiate apoptosis by restoring cellular energy[1]
Apraxia(失用症)	A defect in the understanding of complex motor commands and in the execution of certain learned movements, i.e., deficits in the cognitive components of learned movements[2]
Apraxia(失用症)	在复杂运动指令的理解和在某些已学习动作的执行方面的缺陷，如在认知已学习运动的成分的缺陷[2]
Arcuate scotoma(弧形暗点)	Arcuate scotoma[2]
Arcuate scotoma(弧形暗点)	弧形的暗点[2]
Arnadóttir OT ADL Neurobehavioral Evaluation(Arnadottir OT ADL神经行为评估)	The Árnadóttir OT-ADL Neurobehavioral Evaluation (A-ONE) is a standardized assessment that links performance in activities of daily living (ADL) to neurobehavioral impairments[1]
Arterial embolism(动脉栓塞)	An embolus is a blood clot, bit of tissue or tumor, gas bubble, or other foreign body that circulates in the blood stream until it becomes stuck in a blood vessel[1]
Artery-to-artery embolism(动脉-动脉栓塞)	Thrombus formation on atherosclerotic plaques may embolize to intracranial arteries producing an artery to artery embolic stroke[1]

续　表

英文术语（中文术语）	定义（英文和/或中文）
ASCO Phenotypic System(Asco 表型系统)	The A-S-C-O (phenotypic) classification assigns a graded level of certainty (range 1 to 3) for the presence of each of 4 stroke mechanism categories: atherothrombosis (A), small vessel disease (S), cardio-embolism (C), and other causes (O). This combines etiologic information for individual patients in a single code, which can be grouped according to most likely mechanism (eg, high-risk [C1] cardioembolic source) or any occurrence of a shared phenotype (eg, all cases with evidence for atherosclerosis [A1+A2+A3]). ASCO also includes information on extent of diagnostic evaluation (eg, A0 denotes that no evidence of atherosclerosis was found despite appropriate investigation, whereas A9 signifies that appropriate investigations were not undertaken)[1]
Ascorbic acid(维生素 C)	A six carbon compound related to glucose. It is found naturally in citrus fruits and many vegetables. Ascorbic acid is an essential nutrient in human diets, and necessary to maintain connective tissue and bone. Its biologically active form, vitamin C, functions as a reducing agent and coenzyme in several metabolic pathways. Vitamin C is considered an antioxidant[1]
Asomatognosia(躯体失认症)	Disturbance in the normal awareness of one's own body, typically characterized by one or more of the following symptoms: (1) a tendency to ignore or neglect one side of the body, (2) a failure to recognize or difficulty in identifying a specific part of the body (usually a limb or part of a limb), (3) difficulty in differentiating the right from the left side of the body, or (4) recognizing an impairment in a part of the body (anosognosia)[1]
Aspirin(阿司匹林)	Aspirin blocks prostaglandin synthetase action, which in turn inhibits prostaglandin synthesis and prevents the formation of platelet-aggregating thromboxane A2[1]
Assessment of Motor and Process Skills(运动和过程技能评估)	The Assessment of Motor and Process Skills (AMPS) is an observational assessment widely used by occupational therapists used to measure ADL motor and ADL process skill performance within activities of daily living (ADL)[1]

英文术语（中文术语）	定义（英文和/或中文）
Astasia(站立不能)	Astasia means inability to maintain standing and abasia refers to impaired coordination of gait. The term is usually applied to unusual, often bizarre patterns of gait and stance that appear to have no neuropathophysiologic basis[1]
Asterixis(扑翼样震颤)	Unilateral asterixis has been reported with contralateral lesions involving any possible structure involved in motion (fronto-parietal cortex, basal ganglia, cerebellum, thalamus, brainstem, but not yet in the spinal cord), and exceptionally in ipsilateral brainstem lesion[1]
Asynergia(共济失调)	A type of "dyssynergy" (HP:0010867) characterized by the lack of the ability to smoothly perform the elements of a voluntary movement in the appropriate order and speed[2]
Asynergia(共济失调)	一种类型的"协调障碍"（HP:0010867），特点是缺乏以适当的顺序和速度平稳进行随意运动的能力[2]
Ataxic hemiparesis(震颤性轻偏瘫)	Ataxic hemiparesis is a well-recognized lacunar syndrome involving homolateral ataxia with accompanying corticospinal tract impairment[1]
Ataxic hemiparesis(震颤性轻偏瘫)	Hemiparesis is associated with homolateral ataxia[1]
Ataxic hemiparesis(震颤性轻偏瘫)	Pure motor hemiparesis and ataxic hemiparesis are most frequently due to an infarct in the internal capsule, corona radiata or basis pontis. The deficit is usually proportional, involving face, arm and leg to the same extent[1]
Atherosclerotic Cerebrovascular Disease team(动脉粥样硬化性脑血管病小组)	This is another concept borrowed from trauma care. In larger hospitals, when a severely traumatized patient arrives in the ED, for example after a severe car crash, a team of physicians, nurses, and other healthcare providers collect and work collaboratively to rapidly assess and treat the patient. This same concept is now being applied to stroke victims[1]

续　表

英文术语（中文术语）	定义（英文和/或中文）
Atrial fibrillation(心房颤动)	The most common cause of embolism occurs in a heart (cardiac) condition called "atrial fibrillation." Normally, each electrical impulse causes the atria (upper chambers of the heart) to beat in a strong, coordinated, and efficient manner. The blood flows smoothly. In atrial fibrillation, there are no coordinated electrical impulses, and therefore there is no coordinated mechanical pumping of blood in the atria. When this occurs over long periods of time (usually weeks to months or even longer), clots form in these upper chambers of the heart[1]
Atrial natriuretic factor(心房利钠因子)	The identification of the gene for ANF as a putative candidate gene is consistent with the known circulatory effects of the factor and the finding of elevated levels of ANF in acute ischaemic stroke[1]
Auditory agnosia(听觉失认)	Auditory agnosia refers to impaired perception restricted to certain classes of sounds. For example, word (or verbal) deafness, the most striking type of auditory agnosia, is the incapacity to recognize speech sounds[1]
Auditory hallucinations(幻听)	Phonism is a illusory perception appeared in the auditory illusory which is one of the common symptoms of mental patients, especially in schizophrenia.actually,there is no external acoustic stimulation to the auditory organ[2]
Auditory hallucinations(幻听)	幻听是出现于听觉器官的虚幻的知觉，是精神病人常见症状之一。尤其多见于精神分裂症，而实际上并没有相应的外部声刺激作用于听觉器官[2]
augmentative and alternative communication system(增强交替交流促进疗法)	为言语或重度沟通障碍者设计交流策略和帮助系统的训练方法。常见的有文字、图片、符号交流板、便携式电子交流器等。可用于存在重度言语表达、阅读、书写、手势障碍者达到与对方进行沟通的目的[3]
Axial dystonia(轴向肌张力障碍)	A type of dystonia that affects the midline muscles, i.e., the chest, abdominal, and back muscles[2]
Axial dystonia(轴向肌张力障碍)	一种影响中线肌肉的肌张力障碍，例如胸部、腹部和背部肌肉[2]

英文术语（中文术语）	定义（英文和/或中文）
B-type natriuretic peptide(B型脑钠肽)	A PEPTIDE that is secreted by the BRAIN and the HEART ATRIA, stored mainly in cardiac ventricular MYOCARDIUM. It can cause NATRIURESIS; DIURESIS; VASODILATION; and inhibits secretion of RENIN and ALDOSTERONE. It improves heart function. It contains 32 AMINO ACIDS[1]
Balint syndrome(巴林特综合征)	The Balint syndrome is characterised by : simultanagnosia (inability to perceive more than one object at a time) optic ataxia oculomotor apraxia It typically results from damage to the parieto-occipital regions, and has been associated with : corticobasal degeneration posterior cortical atrophy bilateral parietal ischaemic stroke[1]
Barbiturate(巴比妥盐)	The main effect of barbiturates consists of a decrease in cerebral metabolism. Reduced metabolic rate and subsequent reduction of cerebral blood volume and cerebral blood flow may theoretically reduce edema formation and lower ICP[1]
Barthel Index(Barthel指数)	The Barthel Index measures the individual's performance on 10 ADL functions i.e. feeding, bathing, grooming, dressing, bowel control, bladder control, toileting, chair transfer, ambulation and stair climbing. The index was developed for use in rehabilitation patients with stroke and other neuromuscular or musculoskeletal disorders[1]
Basilar artery infarction syndrome(基底动脉梗死综合征)	The BA lies on the ventral surface of the brainstem and vascularizes the pons, the mesencephalon and the middle and upper cerebellum through the AICA and SCA. Its territory can be subdivided into three parts on a ventro-dorsal level[1]
Behavior compensation strategy(行为补偿)	又称"补偿性策略"。使用适应性设备，用于补偿已丧失的认知或躯体功能的方法。也用于加强被弱化的技能和发展新技能从而使使用者尽可能独立[3]
Behavioral disturbance(行为异常)	Infarction in the mesial frontal lobe can cause psychiatric symptoms, such as emotional lability, euphoria, paralogia, or witzelsucht. Restlessness, hyperactivity, anxiety, agitation, and talkativeness are also common among patients with unilateral caudate infarction. Patients with left-sided caudate lesions have shown a high frequency of severe depression. These behavioural and psychiatric disorders have suggested disturbances of frontocaudate circuits[1]

续　表

英文术语（中文术语）	定义（英文和/或中文）
Behavioral Inattention Test(行为学忽略测试)	The Behavioral Inattention Test (BIT) is a standardized assessment for unilateral visual neglect. It comprises six conventional and nine behavioral subtests[1]
Bell's palsy(Bell麻痹)	Several conditions can cause a facial paralysis, e.g. brain tumor, stroke, and Lyme disease. However, if no specific cause can be identified, the condition is known as Bell's palsy. Named after Scottish anatomist Charles Bell, who first described it. Bell's palsy is the most common acute mononeuropathy (disease involving only one nerve) and is the most common cause of acute facial nerve paralysis. Facial nerve palsy is a dysfunction of cranial nerve VII (the facial nerve) that results in inability to control facial muscles on the affected side with weakness of the muscles of facial expression and eye closure. This can either be present in unilateral or bilateral form[1]
Benedikt syndrome(Benedikt综合征)	Benedikt syndrome, or paramedian midbrain syndrome, is a midbrain stroke syndrome that involves the fascicles of the oculomotor nerve and the red nucleus resulting in an ipsilateral CN III palsy and crossed hemiataxia and chorea. Using imaging alone, it is difficult to distinguish Benedikt from Weber syndrome, unless clear involvement of the red nucleus can be identified, which is seen in the former[1]
Beta carotene intake(β胡萝卜素摄入量)	Beta-carotene, is the biologically active metabolite of vitamin A[1]
Beta globin DNA(β球蛋白DNA)	Circulating levels of DNA measured in plasma increase in response to a variety of injurious conditions, including stroke. Plasma concentration of DNA is elevated within 3 h of ischemic and hemorrhagic stroke onset, and patients who experience a poor outcome or die as a result of their stroke have higher levels than those who do not. The level of DNA also correlates to the volume of hematoma in ICH[1]

英文术语（中文术语）	定义（英文和/或中文）
Beta thromboglobulin(β凝血球蛋白)	A platelet-specific protein which is released when platelets aggregate. Elevated plasma levels have been reported after deep venous thrombosis, pre-eclampsia, myocardial infarction with mural thrombosis, and myeloproliferative disorders. Measurement of beta-thromboglobulin in biological fluids by radioimmunoassay is used for the diagnosis and assessment of progress of thromboembolic disorders [1]
Bilateral ptosis(双侧上睑下垂)	Bilateral ptosis [2]
Bilateral ptosis(双侧上睑下垂)	双侧眼睑的下垂 [2]
Bilateral weakness(双侧无力)	Weakness affecting both sides of the body is not common following a stroke. It may be caused by spinal-cord, bilateral hemispheric, or brainstem infarcts [1]
Binasal hemianopia(双鼻侧偏盲)	Binasal hemianopia [2]
Binasal hemianopia(双鼻侧偏盲)	双眼鼻侧视野缺损 [2]
Binswanger disease(皮层下白质脑病)	Binswanger's disease (BD) is a type of subcortical vascular dementia caused by widespread, microscopic damage to cerebral white matter. The damage is usually the result of atherosclerosis (i.e., narrowing of arterial blood vessels) that reduces the supply of blood to subcortical areas of the brain, causing tissue to die [1]
biofeedback therapy(生物反溃治疗)	将患者意识不到的体内功能活动所产生的信息，通过专门的仪器加以收集、放大并转变为声、光、图像、曲线等信号，使患者得以了解自身的机体状态，从而训练患者对体内异常的不随意生理活动进行自我调节控制以治疗疾病的方法 [3]
Biomarkers in the diagnosis of Atherosclerotic Cerebrovascular Disease(诊断动脉粥样硬化性脑血管病的生物标志物)	A biomarker is any measurable physiological characteristic or substance that marks the risk for or manifestation of a stroke-related process [1]
Bitemporal hemianopia(双颞侧偏盲)	Bitemporal hemianopia [2]
Bitemporal hemianopia(双颞侧偏盲)	双颞侧偏盲 [2]
Blepharospasm(眼睑痉挛)	A focal dystonia that affects the muscles of the eyelids and brow, associated with involuntary recurrent spasm of both eyelids [2]

续　表

英文术语（中文术语）	定义（英文和/或中文）
Blepharospasm(眼睑痉挛)	影响眼睑和额头的肌肉局部肌张力障碍，伴有双眼睑不自主复发性痉挛[2]
Blind-spot enlargment(生理盲点扩大)	Blind-spot enlargment[2]
Blind-spot enlargment(生理盲点扩大)	盲点扩大[2]
blood pressure biofeedback therapy(血压生物反馈疗法)	将专用血压计所测得的血压值动态变化描记为曲线，通过训练患者学会根据曲线所示血压的变化随意调节血压的治疗方法。用于高血压病[3]
Boston Diagnostic Aphasia Examination(波士顿诊断性失语症检查)	The Boston Diagnostic Aphasia Examination (BDAE) is a comprehensive, multiple subtests instrument for investigating a broad range of language impairments that are common consequences of brain damage. It is designed as a comprehensive measure of aphasia. The examination provides materials and procedures to evaluate five language-related sections and an additional section on praxis. The five language domains include conversational and expository speech, auditory comprehension, oral expression, reading, and writing. In addition to individual subtest scores, the test yields three broader measures: the Severity Rating Scale (a rating of the severity of observed language/speech disturbance), the Rating Scale Profile of Speech Characteristics (a rating of observed speech characteristics and of scores in two main language domains), and the Language Competency Index (a composite score of language performance on BDAE-3 subtests)[1]
Box and Block Test(箱块试验)	The Box and Block Test is a simpler measure; it counts the number of blocks that can be transported from one compartment of a box to another compartment within 1 min and is a measure of gross manual dexterity. It can be used with a wide range of populations, including clients with stroke[1]
Brain abscess(脑脓肿)	Brain abscesses are an intracranial mass of immune cells, pus (i.e., collection of dead neutrophils), and other materials stemming from a bacterial or fungal infection[1]
Brain tumor(脑肿瘤)	An abnormal mass of tissue in which some cells (glial or non-glial) grow and multiply uncontrollably. A tumor can be benign or malignant[1]

英文术语（中文术语）	定义（英文和/或中文）
Brain type fatty acid binding protein(脑型脂肪酸结合蛋白)	B-FABP is thought to be present only in central nervous tissue and is undetectable in the serum of healthy individuals [1]
Brainstem infarct syndrome(脑干梗死综合征)	Brainstem stroke syndromes refer to a group of syndromes that occur secondary to occlusion of small perforating arteries of the posterior circulation. The resulted infarction has characteristic clinical picture according to the involved area however, generally there is ipsilateral cranial nerve palsy and contralateral hemiplegia/hemiparesis and sensory loss [1]
Broca aphasia(Broca失语)	This is defined as effortful speech output with hesitations, pauses, word-finding difficulty, phonemic errors (verbal apraxia) consisting of substitutions, deletions, transpositions and anticipations, occasional semantic errors, and agrammatism, but relatively preserved comprehension [1]
Buccofacial apraxia(颊面失用症)	This is an impairment in skilled purposive execution of bucco-lingual and facial movements. As for limb apraxia, testing should assess meaningful, transitive and nontransitive, and meaningless movements involving the lips, tongue, face, or eyelids [1]
C reactive protein(C反应蛋白)	C-reactive protein (CRP) is an acute-phase protein associated with inflammation. Produced in the liver in response to IL-6, CRP binds and aggregates a variety of soluble ligands and activates the classical complement pathway [1]
Calpain 1(钙蛋白酶1)	Calpain 1 is a calcium-activated protease that has been specifically linked to glutamate receptors in the rat hippocampus. It is a mediators facilitate apoptotic cell death pathways [1]
Canadian neurological scale(加拿大神经量表)	The Canadian Neurological Scale (CNS) was designed to monitor mentation and motor functions in stroke patients [1]
Capillary malformation arteriovenous malformation(毛细血管畸形动静脉畸形)	This syndrome is characterised by the association of multiple capillary malformations (CM) with an arteriovenous malformation (AVM) and arteriovenous fistulas [1]
Capsular warning syndrome(内囊预警综合征)	If a severe hemiplegia alternates repeatedly with normal function, the phenomenon is called "capsular warning syndrome", resulting usually from a lacune in the internal capsule [1]

145

续　表

英文术语（中文术语）	定义（英文和/或中文）
Carotenoids(类胡萝卜素)	The general name for a group of fat-soluble pigments found in green, yellow, and leafy vegetables, and yellow fruits. They are aliphatic hydrocarbons consisting of a polyisoprene backbone [1]
Carotid artery atherosclerosis(颈动脉粥样硬化)	Therosclerosis within the carotid artery occures most frequently whithin the common carotid bifurcation and proximal internal carotid artery [1]
Carotid artery dissection(颈动脉夹层)	Dissection of the carotid artery in the neck is a relatively common condition. Most dissections are spontaneous, likely related to activities that cause sudden stretch of the pharyngeal portion of the carotid artery. Carotid artery dissection is a separation of the layers of the artery wall supplying oxygen-bearing blood to the head and brain and is the most common cause of stroke in young adults [1]
Carotid Duplex ultrasound(颈部血管彩超)	Color flow guided duplex ultrasound is well established as a noninvasive examination to evaluate extracranial atherosclerotic disease. This topic is discussed separately [1]
Carotid endarterectomy(颈动脉内膜剥脱术)	Carotid endarterectomy is a surgical procedure to unblock a carotid artery. Carotid endarterectomy is the most frequently performed noncardiac vascular procedure. Recent randomized prospective clinical trials have clearly showed that carotid endarterectomy is a highly beneficial treatment modality compared with the best medical treatment for patients with hemispheric and retinal TIAs or nondisabling strokes and ipsilateral high-grade stenosis of the internal carotid artery [1]
Carotid Intima Media Thickness(颈动脉内膜增厚)	A measurement of the thickness of the carotid artery walls. It is measured by B-mode ULTRASONOGRAPHY and is used as a surrogate marker for ATHEROSCLEROSIS [1]
Carotid sinus syncope［颈动脉窦性晕厥(颈性晕厥)］	An exaggerated response to carotid sinus baroreceptor stimulation resulting in syncope from transient diminished cerebral perfusion [2]
Carotid sinus syncope［颈动脉窦性晕厥(颈性晕厥)］	对颈动脉窦压力感受器的过度反应，导致脑灌注暂时减少，引起晕厥 [2]

英文术语（中文术语）	定义（英文和/或中文）
Carotid siphon atherosclerosis(颈动脉虹吸部动脉粥样硬化)	The carotic siphon (portion whithin the cavernous sinus) is vulnerable to atherosclerosis. Atherosclerosis within the carotid artery occures most frequently whithin the common carotid bifurcation and proximal internal carotid artery [1]
Cathepsin B(组织蛋白酶B)	is a mediators facilitate apoptotic cell death pathways [1]
Catherine Bergego Scale(Catherine Bergego 量表)	The Catherine Bergego Scale (CBS) is based on a direct observation of the patient's functioning in 10 real-life situations, such as grooming, dressing, or wheelchair driving [1]
Causative Classification System(缺血性卒中病因分类系统)	The CCS scheme also assigns patients into 5 mechanism-based categories: cardio-aortic, large artery atherosclerosis, small artery occlusion, other cause, and undetermined. However, unlike TOAST, the CCS system assigns the most likely subtype based on updated estimates of stroke risks associated with specific cardiac and vascular pathologies or clinical or imaging parameters known to be more commonly associated with particular stroke mechanisms [1]
Cavernous angioma(海绵状血管瘤)	A cavernous angioma is a blood vessel abnormality characterized by large, adjacent capillaries with little or no intervening brain. The blood flow through these vessels is slow [1]
CC chemokine receptor 2(CC趋化因子受体 2)	CCR receptors with specificity for CHEMOKINE CCL2 and several other CCL2-related chemokines. They are expressed at high levels in T-LYMPHOCYTES; B-LYMPHOCYTES; MACROPHAGES; BASOPHILS; and NK CELLS [1]
CC chemokine receptor 7(CC趋化因子受体 7)	CCR7 is a G-coupled chemokine receptor and the data on CCR7 function in humans are rather sparse [1]
CC chemokine receptors(CC趋化因子受体)	Chemokine receptors that are specific for CC CHEMOKINES [1]

续　表

英文术语（中文术语）	定义（英文和/或中文）
Cell death(细胞死亡)	Any biological process that results in permanent cessation of all vital functions of a cell. A cell should be considered dead when any one of the following molecular or morphological criteria is met: (1) the cell has lost the integrity of its plasma membrane; (2) the cell, including its nucleus, has undergone complete fragmentation into discrete bodies (frequently referred to as "apoptotic bodies"); and/or (3) its corpse (or its fragments) have been engulfed by an adjacent cell in vivo [1]
Cell death(细胞死亡)	The most satisfactory definition of cell death, and the one that would be the most valuable to know therapeutically, is the point at which the cell becomes unable to recover its normal morphology and function even if all processes leading to dissoution are stopped pharmacologically (the point of no return) [1]
Central scotoma(中心暗点)	An area of depressed vision located at the point of fixation and that interferes with central vision [2]
Central scotoma(中心暗点)	视物时视野中央部存在暗区并干扰中央视觉 [2]
Centrocaecal scotoma(近中心性暗点)	A scotoma (area of diminished vision within the visual field) located between the central point of fixation and the blind spot with a roughly horizontal oval shape [2]
Centrocaecal scotoma(近中心性暗点)	盲点（视觉范围内视力消失的区域）位于中心点与生理盲点之间大致水平的椭圆形区域内 [2]
Cerebellar ataxia associated with quadrupedal gait(小脑性共济失调与四足步态相关)	The presence of cerebellar signs and symptoms such as lack of balance associated with quadrupedal gait (locomotion on all four extremities with a 'bear-like' gait with the legs held straight) [2]
Cerebellar ataxia associated with quadrupedal gait(小脑性共济失调与四足步态相关)	出现小脑的症状和体征，如缺乏平衡与四足步态相关（所有四肢以"熊样"步态运动，腿部保持笔直）[2]
Cerebellar infarction syndrome(小脑梗死综合征)	Cerebellar infarction is a relatively uncommon subtype of ischaemic stroke. It may involve any of the three arteries supplying the cerebellum: -superior cerebellar artery (SCA): superior cerebellar arterial infarct -anterior inferior cerebellar artery (AICA): anterior inferior cerebellar arterial infarct -posterior inferior cerebellar artery (PICA): posterior inferior cerebellar arterial infarct [1]

英文术语（中文术语）	定义（英文和/或中文）
Cerebral edema(脑水肿)	Expansion of the size of the brain that occurs following head trauma and brain injury[1]
Cerebral venous sinus thrombosis(颅内静脉窦血栓形成)	Cerebral venous sinus thrombosis (CVST) is a rare and potentially deadly condition. Common etiologies include hypercoagulable diseases, low flow states, dehydration, adjacent infectious processes, oral contraceptives, hormonal replacement therapy, pregnancy, and puerperium. Symptoms include nausea, seizures, severe focal neurological deficits, coma, and headache (the most common presenting symptom)[1]
Cerebral venous thrombosis(颅内静脉系统血栓形成)	Cerebral venous thrombosis is an infrequent condition characterized by extreme variability in its clinical presentation and mode of onset[1]
cerebrovascular spasm(脑血管痉挛)	Cerebral vasospasm may lead to permanent neurologic deficits of fatal cerebral edema. It appears to be mediated principally by the vascular musculature, but intrinsic neurogenic reflex activity may also play a part, as may control by an extrinsic innervation of the cerebral arteries[1]
Cervical artery dissection(颈部动脉夹层)	Arterial dissection is an uncommon vascular wall condition that typically involves a tear at some point in the artery's lining and the formation of an intimal flap, which allows blood to penetrate into the muscular portion of the vessel wall[1]
Charlson Comorbidity Index(察尔森合并症指数)	The Charlson Comorbidity Index (CCI) has been validated for ischaemic stroke outcome studies. However, it was originally developed for patients in acute hospital settings, and it focused on mortality, not functional impairment[1]
Chedoke Arm and Hand Activity Inventory(切多克手臂和手部活动清单)	The CAHAI consists of 13 real-life functional tasks that reflect (1) the domains deemed important by survivors of stroke; (2) bilateral activities; (3) non-gender-specific items; (4) the full range of normative movements, pinches, and grasps; and (5) the various stages of motor recovery poststroke[1]

续　表

英文术语（中文术语）	定义（英文和/或中文）
Chedoke McMaster Stroke Assessment(切多克·麦克马斯特中风评估)	he Chedoke-McMaster Stroke Assessment measures the physical impairments and disabilities that impact on the lives of individuals with stroke. This measure has three overall purposes: 1) to stage motor recovery to classify individuals in terms of clinical characteristics, 2) to predict rehabilitation outcomes, and 3) to measure clinically important change in physical function [1]
Cheyne-Stokes respiration(潮式呼吸)	This is well known in bihemispheric stroke, heart failure, somnolence, and brain edema with increased intracranial pressure [1]
Chin myoclonus(下颌肌阵挛)	Involuntary and irregular twitches of the chin [2]
Chin myoclonus(下颌肌阵挛)	下巴不自主和不规则抽动 [2]
Chocolate(巧克力)	High consumption of chocolate is associated with a 29% (95% CI 2–48) lower risk of stroke [1]
Chorea(舞蹈病)	Chorea (Greek for 'dance') refers to widespread arrhythmic involuntary movements of a forcible, jerky and restless fashion [2]
Chorea(舞蹈病)	Chorea is characterized by brief, irregular muscle contractions that are not repetitive or rhythmic, but appear to flow from one muscle to the next. They may appear as dance-like movements of the limbs, trunk, or head. Typical movements include facial grimacing, shoulder adduction, and finger extension and contractions. They can be associated with snakelike writhing movements of the hands or feet known as athetosis [1]
Chorea(舞蹈病)	舞蹈样运动（希腊文"跳舞"），指的是广泛无节奏的不自主强行运动，表现为抽动样，坐立不安 [2]
Choreoathetosis(舞蹈手足徐动症)	Involuntary movements characterized by both athetosis (inability to sustain muscles in a fixed position) and chorea (widespread jerky arrhythmic movements) [2]
Choreoathetosis(舞蹈手足徐动症)	以手足徐动（无法维持肌肉在固定位置）和舞蹈样运动（广泛无节奏的不自主强行运动）为特征的不自主运动 [2]
Citicoline(胞二磷胆碱)	Citicoline is an exogenous form of cytidine-5'-diphosphocholine (CDP-choline) used in membrane biosynthesis. Citicoline may reduce ischemic injury by stabilizing membranes and decreasing free radical formation [1]

英文术语（中文术语）	定义（英文和/或中文）
Claude syndrome(克劳德综合征)	Claude syndrome is one of the brainstem stroke syndromes in which there is infarction of the dorsomedial aspect of the midbrain secondary to occlusion of the small perforating branches of the posterior cerebral artery supplying this area. The infarction involves the medial aspect of red nucleus with the rubrodentate fibers, CN III nucleus and superior cerebellar peduncle. Clinical picture is characteristic and includes ipsilateral oculomotor nerve palsy and contralateral upper and lower limb ataxia [1]
Clomethiazole(氯美噻唑)	Clomethiazole, a gamma-aminobutyric acid agonist, decreases excitatory neurotransmission by increasing activity of inhibitory pathways [1]
Clopidogrel(氯吡格雷)	Clopidogrel inhibits platelet aggregation and is used for secondary stroke prevention. It is indicated for the reduction of atherothrombotic events following a recent stroke [1]
Cluster headache(丛集性头痛)	A type of headache characterized by repeated attacks of unilateral pain lasting 15 to 180 minutes and associated with local autonomic signs [2]
Cluster headache(丛集性头痛)	一种单侧反复密集发作的头痛，一般持续15?180分钟，并伴有局部自主神经体征 [2]
Coagulation disorder(凝血障碍)	Disorders involving the elements of blood coagulation, including platelets, coagulation factors and inhibitors, and the fibrinolytic system [1]
Coca alkaloid(可可碱)	Coca alkaloids are the alkaloids found in the coca plant, Erythroxylum coca [1]
Cocaine hydrochloride(可卡因)	Cocaine is a naturally occurring chemical found in the leaves of Erythroxylum coca or coca plant, which is native to South America. Coca leaves have been used and abused for hundreds of years. Cocaine is a highly addictive stimulant drug that directly affects the nervous system, including the brain [1]
Coffee intake(咖啡摄入量)	the consumption of coffee (3–4 cups) has been associated with a reduction in the risk of stroke [1]

151

续　表

英文术语（中文术语）	定义（英文和/或中文）
Cognitive disturbance(认知功能障碍)	Cognitive disturbances consist mostly of personality changes with disinhibited behavior, impulsivity, apathy and even loss of psychic selfactivation associated with amnesia similar to Korsakoff syndrome[1]
Collier's sign(Collier's征)	Collier's sign is well known as unilateral or bilateral eyelid retraction due to midbrain lesions. This sign is usually caused by infarction, tumor, multiple sclerosis, neuro-degenerative disease, or encephalitis[1]
Coma(昏迷)	Coma refers to a sleep-like state of unarousability in which consciousness is completely absent. Comatose patients keep their eyes closed even after painful stimuli, are not capable of any comprehensible verbal response, do not obey commands, and do not localize painful stimuli, although they may make posturing and reflexive responses. The percentage of patients in coma ranges from 5–18% in ischemic stroke to 31–55% in intracerebral hemorrhage (ICH)[1]
Coma(昏迷)	Complete absence of wakefulness and content of conscience, which manifests itself as a lack of response to any kind of external stimuli[2]
Coma(昏迷)	完全没有觉醒和意识内容，表现为对任何外部刺激没有反应[2]
Comorbidity(合并症)	The presence of co-existing or additional diseases with reference to an initial diagnosis or with reference to the index condition that is the subject of study. Comorbidity may affect the ability of affected individuals to function and also their survival; it may be used as a prognostic indicator for length of hospital stay, cost factors, and outcome or survival[1]
Complement C3(补体C3)	Complement C3 plays a key role in the activation of the complement system and in the inflammatory process. Complement activation occurs early in cases of ischemia/reperfusion injury leading to the release of biologically active substances including C3 a-chain and mediates cerebral ischemia/reperfusion injury[1]

英文术语（中文术语）	定义（英文和/或中文）
Complex hyperkinesias(复杂运动过度)	The most complex hyperkinesia associated with stroke is found in association with posterio-lateral thalamic strokes, mostly posterior choroidal or thalamogeniculate. A mixture of rubral tremor, chorea, pseudoathetosis, myoclonus, dystonia and ataxia is regularly found, which has been called the "jerky dystonic unsteady hand syndrome" by our group. When associated with a painful syndrome, this is well known as the Dejerine–Roussy syndrome. Very complex dyskinesia with dystonia, avoidance and withdrawal behaviors, hypertonia (poikilotonia), persistence of awkward postures (hemicatalepsy, levitation), akinesia, multiple apraxias, ataxia, and sensorimotor deficits is found in the parietal lobe motor syndrome, but also in temporo-parietal, basal ganglia and fronto-cingulate strokes (also see maniform agitation, compulsive motor behaviours and athymormic states above)[1]
Complication(并发症)	Medical complications of acute ischemic stroke are common and influence outcome after ischemic stroke[1]
Composite Spasticity Index(综合痉挛指数)	The Composite Spasticity Index (CSI) s a measure of upper and lower extremity spasticity that is suitable for use with patients with hemiparesis following stroke. The CSI measures the phasic stretch reflex by assessing the tendon jerk and clonus, and the tonic stretch reflex with assessment of resistance to passive movement of the limb[1]
Comprehensive stroke center(综合卒中中心)	The CSC is designed to care for patients with complicated types of strokes, patients with intracerebral hemorrhage or subarachnoid hemorrhage, and those requiring specific interventions (eg, surgery or endovascular procedures) or an intensive care unit type of setting[1]
Congenital bilateral ptosis(先天性双侧上睑下垂)	Congenital bilateral ptosis[2]
Congenital bilateral ptosis(先天性双侧上睑下垂)	先天性双眼上睑下垂[2]
Congenital horizontal nystagmus(先天性水平眼震)	Horizontal nystagmus dating from or present at birth[2]

续　表

英文术语（中文术语）	定义（英文和/或中文）
Congenital horizontal nystagmus(先天性水平眼震)	出生后即起病的眼球水平眼震[2]
Congenital Horner syndrome(先天性霍纳综合征)	A type of "Horner syndrome" (HP:0002277) with congenital onset[2]
Congenital Horner syndrome(先天性霍纳综合征)	霍纳综合征的一种 ` (HP:0002277)，先天性发病[2]
Congenital miosis(先天性瞳孔缩小)	Abnormal (non-physiological) constriction of the pupil of congenital onset[2]
Congenital miosis(先天性瞳孔缩小)	先天发病的、异常（非生理的）的瞳孔缩小[2]
Congenital nystagmus(先天性眼球震颤)	Nystagmus dating from or present at birth[2]
Congenital nystagmus(先天性眼球震颤)	出生后即发生的眼球震颤[2]
Congenital ptosis(先天性上睑下垂)	Congenital ptosis[2]
Congenital ptosis(先天性上睑下垂)	先天性上睑下垂[2]
Congruous heteronymous hemianopia(一致性对侧偏盲)	Congruous heteronymous hemianopia[2]
Congruous heteronymous hemianopia(一致性对侧偏盲)	一致性异侧偏盲[2]
Congruous homonymous hemianopia(一致性同侧偏盲)	Congruous homonymous hemianopia[2]
Congruous homonymous hemianopia(一致性同侧偏盲)	一致性同侧偏盲[2]
Conjugate gaze paresis(共轭凝视轻瘫)	Conjugate-gaze palsy is one of the most common eyemovement abnormalities in patients with acute stroke. The eyes may be deviated to one side, either to the side of a hemispheral lesion or to the opposite side of a pons lesion, with gaze paresis towards the opposite side. This gaze palsy is almost invariably accompanied by hemiparesis[1]

英文术语（中文术语）	定义（英文和/或中文）
Consciousness(意识清晰)	The commonplace dictionary definitions of consciousness tend to fare better since they often state that consciousness is the ability to be aware of self and surroundings. These definitions are circular – given that awareness is often seen as a synonym of consciousness itself, or at least as a significant part of it – but in spite of the circularity, such definitions capture something essential: consciousness does allow us to know of our own existence and of the existence of objects and events, inside and outside our organism [1]
Constipation(便秘)	Constipation is recognized as a serious problem in clinical practice, affecting 60% of those in stroke rehabilitation wards [1]
Constricted visual fields(视野狭窄)	Constricted visual fields [2]
Constricted visual fields(视野狭窄)	外周视野缺损导致视野狭窄 [2]
constructional apraxia(结构性失用)	An inability to execute or copy simple drawings (cube, clock, house), or to arrange elements (blocks or sticks) in an appropriate spatial relationship, is a very sensitive sign of brain damage but relatively non-specific. It implicates a number of basic skills, including visual and spatial perception, visuomotor integration and coordination, motor manual skills, and monitoring responses. Therefore, it can result from a variety of lesions, and often indicates coexistent general intellectual deterioration [1]
Contralateral fourth cranial nerve palsy(对侧第四颅神经麻痹)	Paralysis of the fourth cranial (trochlear) nerve manifested as weakness of the superior oblique muscle which causes vertical diplopia that is maximal when the affected eye is adducted and directed inferiorly. The fourth cranial nerve crosses as it exits the midbrain dorsally and may be injured along its course through the intracranial space, cavernous sinus, superior orbital fissure, or orbit [1]
Contralateral hemiplegia(对侧偏瘫)	characteristic presentation of a lesion of the descending motor pathways proximal to the decussation, in which the resulting limb weakness is on the side opposite to the brain lesion [1]

续　表

英文术语（中文术语）	定义（英文和/或中文）
Contralateral hyperkinetic movements(对侧运动过度)	Movements that are either voluntary or involuntary and result in excessive movements. The most common types of hyperkinetic movements are tremor, myoclonus, dystonia, dyskinesias, and tics[1]
Contralateral limb ataxia(对侧肢体共济失调)	A kind of ataxia that affects movements of the extremities. Limb ataxia is generally caused by lesions of the cerebellar hemispheres and associated pathways[1]
Contralateral thermoalgesic deficit(对侧痛温觉减退)	High sensibility to heat; pain caused by a slight degree of heat[1]
contrast bath(冷热交替浴)	将需要治疗的身体部分交替浸入热水与冷水之中，或以热水与冷水交替喷射某一患部进行治疗的方法[3]
Contrast Enhanced MRA(对比增强MRA)	A technique that uses radiofrequency waves and a magnet to image the body. The images are enhanced by the addition of contrast agents which selectively intensify anatomical regions to intensify the clarity of the image for diagnostic purposes[1]
Contrast Enhanced MRA(对比增强MRA)	Contrast-enhanced MRA (CE MRA) is performed with a rapid, short repetition time (TR, 10ms) gradient echo sequence following an i.v. bolus of gadolinium[1]
Conventional angiography(常规血管造影)	Digital subtraction angiography, the most widely used method of conventional catheter-based angiography, remains the gold standard for evaluating the cerebral vessels with regard to determining the degree of arterial stenosis and the presence of dissection, vasculopathy, vasculitis, or occult lesions such as vascular malformations[1]
Cortical blindness syndrome(皮质盲综合征)	Cortical blindness refers to severe visual loss produced by bilateral damage to the geniculostriate visual pathways. The underlying pathophysiological mechanism involves direct destruction and/or de-afferentation of primary visual cortex. The term Anton's syndrome is applied to patients with cortical blindness who demonstrate explicit denial or unawareness (anosognosia) of their visual impairment[1]

英文术语（中文术语）	定义（英文和/或中文）
Cortical deafness(皮层耳聋)	Cortical deafness is a rare condition occurring with bilateral temporal lobe lesions or with bilateral subcortical lesions interrupting the ascending auditory pathways. In cortical deafness, patients appear deaf, though some reflex responses such as turning toward a sudden loud sound may be preserved. With time, some auditory capacities may re-emerge[1]
CR1(补体受体1)	CR1, a novel gene for Alzheimer's disease identified using genome-wide association studies, has also been implicated in intracerebral hemorrhage[1]
Crack cocaine(强效可卡因)	Crack cocaine is the freebase form of cocaine that can be smoked. It may also be termed rock, work, hard, iron, cavvy, base, but is most commonly known as just crack; the Manual of Adolescent Substance Abuse Treatment calls it the most addictive form of cocaine[1]
Craniofacial dystonia(头面部肌张力障碍)	A form of focal dystonia affecting the face, head or neck muscles[2]
Craniofacial dystonia(头面部肌张力障碍)	一种累及面部、头部或颈部肌肉的局限性肌张力障碍[2]
Crossed hemiataxia(交叉性偏身共济失调)	Hemiataxia is a common occurrence in thalamic infarction involving the ventrolateral part of the thalamus usually from involvement of the thalamogeniculate territory[1]
Crossed hemihypesthesia(交叉偏身感觉减退)	Diminished sensibility in one side of the body[1]
cryotherapy(冷疗法)	以寒冷作用于皮肤或黏膜以治疗疾病的方法[3]
Cytotoxic edema(细胞毒性水肿)	Cytotoxic edema is defined as the premorbid cellular process, otherwise known as cellular edema, oncotic cell swelling, or oncosis, whereby extracellular Na+ and other cations enter into neurons and astrocytes and accumulate intracellularly, in part due to failure of energy-dependent mechanisms of extrusion[1]
Dabigatran(达比加群酯)	Dabigatran etexilate is the orally administered prodrug and is rapidly converted by tissue esterases to dabigatran, a direct thrombin inhibitor. When taken by mouth, the bioavailability of dabigatran is approximately 7%[1]
Death(死亡)	The immediate period after an ischemic stroke carries the greatest risk of death, with fatality rates ranging from 8% to 20% in the first 30 days[1]

续　表

英文术语（中文术语）	定义（英文和/或中文）
Deep venous thrombosis(深静脉血栓形成)	Deep-vein thrombosis (DVT) is a common condition that can lead to complications such as postphlebitic syndrome, pulmonary embolism and death[1]
Delirium(谵妄)	Delirium is characterized by reduced ability to maintain attention; disturbance of immediate memory; and disorganized, slowed, and impoverished thinking. Disorientation, altered shortterm and long-term memory, illusions, and hallucinations are frequently but not invariably present. Although delirium usually is accompanied by decreased arousal and psychomotor slowing, occasionally it may be characterized by hypervigilance and enhanced psychomotor activity. Occasionally, there is a "dreamy" or "twilight" state associated with partial loss of contact with the outer world[1]
Depression(抑郁症)	An affective disorder manifested by either a dysphoric mood or loss of interest or pleasure in usual activities. The mood disturbance is prominent and relatively persistent[1]
Deuteranomoly(绿色弱视)	A type of anomalous trichromacy associated with abnormal M photopigment, such that the absorption spectrum is shifted toward L wavelengths. Affected individuals have difficulties distinguishing between red and green[2]
Deuteranomoly(绿色弱视)	异常三色视的一种，M波长感光色素异常，使得吸收光谱移向L波长，患者的红绿色觉异常[2]
Deuteranopia(绿色盲)	Complete lack of the M photopigment, which is replaced with the L photopigment. Affected individuals tend to confuse red and green[2]
Deuteranopia(绿色盲)	完全缺乏M波长感光色素，由L感光色素替代。患者分辨不出红色和绿色[2]
Diabetes mellitus(糖尿病)	A heterogeneous group of disorders characterized by HYPERGLYCEMIA and GLUCOSE INTOLERANCE[1]

英文术语（中文术语）	定义（英文和/或中文）
Diagnosis(诊断)	Diagnosis of a disease or condition made before DEATH. The determination of the nature of a disease or condition, or the distinguishing of one disease or condition from another. Assessment may be made through physical examination, laboratory tests, or the likes. Computerized programs may be used to enhance the decision-making process. Diagnosis of a disease or condition made after DEATH[1]
Diagnosis cost group(诊断费用组)	DCGs were originally developed to predict future costs for Medicare beneficiaries. Each ICD-9-CM code is first grouped into diagnostic clusters of clinically related disorders. Clusters are subsequently grouped into hierarchical condition categories that consider the severity and expected costliness of related disorders. Examples of hierarchies are congestive heart failure and diabetes mellitus with chronic complications. Hierarchies may be further clustered into aggregated condition categories[1]
Diagnostic tests(诊断测试)	Diagnostic procedures, such as laboratory tests and x-rays, routinely performed on all individuals or specified categories of individuals in a specified situation, e.g., patients being admitted to the hospital. These include routine tests administered to neonates[1]
Dichromacy(双色盲)	Individuals affected by dichromacy possess only two types of cones, instead of three[2]
Dichromacy(双色盲)	患者只有两种类型的视锥细胞，而不是通常的三种[2]
Dietary Approaches to Stop Hypertension diet(控制高血压饮食的饮食方法)	The DASH diet is comprised of four to five servings of fruit, four to five servings of vegetables, two to three servings of low-fat dairy per day, and <25 percent dietary intake from fat. The DASH diet has been studied in both normotensive and hypertensive populations and found to lower systolic and diastolic pressure more than a diet rich in fruits and vegetables alone. The combination of low-sodium and DASH diet resulted in further decreases in blood pressure, comparable with those observed with antihypertensive agents[1]

续　表

英文术语（中文术语）	定义（英文和/或中文）
Dietary Approaches to Stop Hypertension diet(控制高血压饮食的饮食方法)	The Dietary Approaches to Stop Hypertension (DASH) diet contains a high intake of plant foods, fruits and vegetables, fi sh, poultry, whole grains, low-fat dairy products, and nuts, while minimising intake of red meat, sodium, sweets, and sugar-sweetened beverages [1]
Dietary factor(饮食因素)	The consideration of dietary factors as a variable in disease incident, transmission, and control [1]
Differential diagnosis(鉴别诊断)	Differential diagnosis refers to the process of differentiating one diagnosis from another, and in turn, providing the most fitting diagnosis based on an individual's presentation [1]
Diffusion weighted magnetic resonance imaging(磁共振弥散加权成像)	Diffusion-weighted MRI (DWI) is highly sensitive in detecting early cerebral ischemic changes in acute stroke patients [1]
Diplopia(复视)	Diplopia is a condition in which a single object is perceived as two images, it is also known as double vision [1]
Dipyridamole with aspirin(阿司匹林双嘧达莫片)	The combination of extended-release dipyridamole and aspirin reduces the relative risk of stroke, death, and myocardial infarction (MI). It is used for the secondary prevention of ischemic stroke and TIAs [1]
Disability Assessment Scale(残疾评估量表)	Disability Assessment Scale (DAS) was developed to assess functional impairment commonly seen in patients with poststroke upper-limb spasticity (ie, dressing, hygiene, limb position, pain) [1]
disruption of Brain blood barrier(血脑屏障破坏)	Loss of integrity of the blood–brain barrier (BBB) resulting from ischemia [1]
Dissociated nystagmus(分离性眼震)	Divergence nystagmus [2]
Dissociated nystagmus(分离性眼震)	散开性眼震 [2]
Distal limb weakness (下肢远端无力)	Motor deficits are among the most common manifestations in patients with ACA-territory infarctions. In classic descriptions, cortical branch occlusion usually results in motor deficits of the foot and leg and, to a lesser degree, paresis of the arm, with the face and tongue largely spared. Leg weakness is most severe distally [1]

英文术语（中文术语）	定义（英文和/或中文）
Downbeat nystagmus(下跳性眼球震颤)	Downbeat nystagmus is a type of fixation nystagmus with the fast phase beating in a downward direction. It generally increases when looking to the side and down and when lying prone [2]
Downbeat nystagmus(下跳性眼球震颤)	下击型眼球震颤是指向下方的快相跳动的眼球震颤。向侧面看、向下看或躺下时症状加重 [2]
Dysarthria clumsy hand syndrome(构音困难手笨拙综合征)	Dysarthria–clumsy hand syndrome is due most of the time to a lacunar infarct in the basis pontis, less frequently to a lesion in the internal capsule or cerebral peduncle [1]
Dyschromatopsia(色觉障碍)	A form of colorblindness in which only two of the three fundamental colors can be distinguished due to a lack of one of the retinal cone pigments [2]
Dyschromatopsia(色觉障碍)	dyschromatopsia is a form of loss of color perception [1]
Dyschromatopsia(色觉障碍)	色盲的一种形式，色觉障碍患者由于缺乏一种视锥细胞色素，只能识别三种基本色中的两种 [2]
Dysdiadochokinesis(轮替运动障碍)	A type of "ataxia" (HP:0001251) characterized by the impairment of the ability to perform rapidly alternating movements, such as rhythmically tapping the fingers on the knee, generally related to a cerebellar lesion [2]
Dysdiadochokinesis(轮替运动障碍)	"共济失调"（HP:0001251）的表现之一，表现为进行快速交替运动的功能受损，比如不能有节奏地用手拍打膝盖，一般为小脑病变所致 [2]
Dysesthesia(感觉迟钝)	Abnormal sensations with no apparent physical cause that are painful or unpleasant [2]
Dysesthesia(感觉迟钝)	没有明显物理原因而存在异常的疼痛或不愉快的感觉 [2]
Dyslipidemia(脂蛋白代谢紊乱)	Abnormalities in the serum levels of LIPIDS, including overproduction or deficiency. Abnormal serum lipid profiles may include high total CHOLESTEROL, high TRIGLYCERIDES, low HIGH DENSITY LIPOPROTEIN CHOLESTEROL, and elevated LOW DENSITY LIPOPROTEIN CHOLESTEROL [1]
Dysmetria(辨距不良)	A type of "ataxia" (HP:0001251) characterized by the inability to carry out movements with the correct range and motion across the plane of more than one joint related to incorrect estimation of the distances required for targeted movements [2]

续　表

英文术语（中文术语）	定义（英文和/或中文）
Dysmetria(辨距不良)	"共济失调"（HP:0001251）的一种，表现为因对完成目标动作需要的距离估计错误，导致不能在正确的范围内执行运动[2]
Dysphagia(吞咽障碍)	Difficulty in swallowing[2]
Dysphagia(吞咽障碍)	In the context of stroke, oropharyngeal dysphagia is probably best defined as a disruption of bolus flow through the mouth and pharynx[1]
Dysphagia(吞咽障碍)	ysphagia is a common complication of stroke and is a major risk factor for developing aspiration pneumonia[1]
Dysphagia(吞咽障碍)	吞咽困难[2]
Dysphonia(发声困难)	An impairment in the ability to produce voice sounds[2]
Dysphonia(发声困难)	产生声音的能力减弱[2]
Dyspraxia(失用)	Alien hand syndrome (AHS) is a relatively rare manifestation of damage to specific brain regions involved in voluntary movement[1]
Dyssynergia(协同失调)	A type of "ataxia" (HP:0001251) characterized by the impairment of the ability to smoothly perform the elements of a voluntary movement in the appropriate order and speed. With dyssynergia, a voluntary movement appears broken down into its component parts[2]
Dyssynergia(协同失调)	"共济失调"（HP:0001251)的一种，表现为按照适当的顺序和速度进行的随意运动能力受损。协调失调时，随意运动表现为它的组成部分的分解动作[2]
Dystonia(肌张力障碍综合征)	An abnormally increased muscular tone that causes fixed abnormal postures. There is a slow, intermittent twisting motion that leads to exaggerated turning and posture of the extremities and trunk[2]

英文术语（中文术语）	定义（英文和/或中文）
Dystonia(肌张力障碍综合征)	Dystonia is defined as a persistent inappropriate posture at rest or on action, in overflexion, overextension or rotation by prolonged cocontraction of antagonist muscles or simply tonic contraction of focal muscles (dystonic posture), sometimes associated with various movements (dystonic movements) such as tremor like jerky motion (dystonic tremor) or athetotic snake-like movements (athetotic dystonia or athetosis), or muscle jerks (dystonic myoclonus)[1]
Dystonia(肌张力障碍综合征)	肌张力异常增加导致固定的异常姿势。因为缓慢和间歇的扭转运动导致四肢和躯干的夸张旋转和姿势[2]
Edoxaban(艾多沙班)	Edoxaban, an oral direct factor Xa inhibitor, has been found non-inferior to warfarin for preventing stroke and systemic embolism in patients with non-valvular atrial fibrillation (NVAF), with a lower rate of intracranial bleeding[1]
electroencepha-lographic biofeedback therapy(脑电生物反馈疗法)	通过脑电信号反馈进行治疗的方法。用于抑郁症、神经症、失眠、癫痫等[3]
Electroencephalography(脑电图)	Recording of electric currents developed in the brain by means of electrodes applied to the scalp, to the surface of the brain, or placed within the substance of the brain[1]
electromyographic biofeedback therapy(肌电生物反馈疗法)	通过肌电信号反馈进行治疗的方法。用于增强肌力训练、放松肌肉训练、紧张性头痛等[3]
Electrophysiological biomarkers of stroke(脑卒中的电生理生物标志物)	Electrophysiology holds both practical and theoretical advantages as a clinical biomarker in neurodevelopmental disorders[1]
Endothelial dysfunction(内皮功能障碍)	In vascular diseases, endothelial dysfunction is a systemic pathological state of the endothelium (the inner lining of blood vessels) and can be broadly defined as an imbalance between vasodilating and vasoconstricting substances produced by (or acting on) the endothelium. Normal functions of endothelial cells include mediation of coagulation, platelet adhesion, immune function and control of volume and electrolyte content of the intravascular and extravascular spaces. Endothelial dysfunction is a risk factor for cerebrovascular events[1]

续　表

英文术语（中文术语）	定义（英文和/或中文）
Endovascular Interventions(血管内介入治疗)	Several endovascular interventions are being evaluated for the treatment of intracranial or extracranial arterial occlusions leading to acute ischemic stroke. Options include emergency angioplasty and stenting, mechanical disruption of the clot, and extraction of the thrombus. In most cases, the mechanical intervention has been combined with either intravenous or intra-arterial thrombolytic therapy[1]
Ephedrine(麻黄碱)	Ephedrine is a sympathomimetic amine and substituted amphetamine commonly used as a stimulant, concentration aid, decongestant, appetite suppressant, and to treat hypotension associated with anaesthesia[1]
Epidural bleeding(硬膜外出血)	Bleeding between the skull and the dura, the thick, outermost layer covering the brain[1]
Epilepsy(癫痫)	The risk of epilepsy following stroke for the individualis low,about3%,yet still higher than the age-matched population[1]
Epileptic seizure(癫痫发作)	Seizures following stroke are common and occur in about 9% of patients overall, especially in the first few weeks. Seizures aremorecommonafter cerebral hemorrhage than infarction[1]
Episodic ataxia(发作性共济失调)	Periodic spells of incoordination and imbalance[2]
Episodic ataxia(发作性共济失调)	周期性发作的不协调和不平衡[2]
Episodic quadriplegia(阵发性全瘫)	Intermittent episodes of paralysis of all four limbs[2]
Episodic quadriplegia(阵发性全瘫)	间歇性发作的四肢瘫痪[2]
Episodic vomiting(阵发性呕吐)	Paroxysmal, recurrent episodes of vomiting[2]
Episodic vomiting(阵发性呕吐)	阵发性、反复发作的呕吐[2]
Estrogen replacement therapy(雌激素替代治疗)	The use of hormonal agents with estrogen-like activity in postmenopausal or other estrogen-deficient women to alleviate effects of hormone deficiency, such as vasomotor symptoms, DYSPAREUNIA, and progressive development of OSTEOPOROSIS. This may also include the use of progestational agents in combination therapy[1]
Euphoria(欣快)	An exaggerated state of psychological and physical well being[1]

英文术语（中文术语）	定义（英文和/或中文）
Evaluation of Atherosclerotic Cerebrovascular Disease(动脉粥样硬化性脑血管病评价)	An overview of the evaluation of patients who present with neurologic symptoms that may be consistent with stroke includes the following: understanding the classification of stroke, An initial quick evaluation to stabilize vital signs, determine if intracranial hemorrhage is present, and, in patients with ischemic stroke, decide if reperfusion therapy is warranted, Forming a hypothesis of the stroke etiology based upon the history, physical examination, and initial brain imaging study (usually a noncontrast head CT scan) and Confirming the precise pathophysiologic process with more directed diagnostic testing[1]
Excitotoxicity(兴奋性细胞毒作用)	The pathological process by which nerve cells are damaged and killed by excessive stimulation by neurotransmitters such as glutamate and similar substances. (Source: http://en.wikipedia.org/wiki/Excitotoxicity)[1]
Eyelid apraxia(眼睑失用症)	Eyelid apraxia is manifested as involuntary levator muscle suppression and orbicularis oculi muscle inhibition. It is one of the typical signs of Parkinson's disease in the elderly[2]
F2 isoprostanes(F2异前列腺素)	F2-isoprostanes (F2IPs) are prostaglandin-like products of noncyclooxygenase free radical–induced peroxidation of arachidonic acid[1]
Facial colliculus syndrome(面丘综合征)	Facial colliculus syndrome refers to a constellation of neurological signs due to a lesion at the facial colliculus, involving: abducens nerve (CN VI) nucleus, facial nerve (CN VII) fibres at the genu and medial longitudinal fasciculus[1]
Facial paralysis(面瘫)	Facial paralysis can be caused by compression of the facial nerve.The main difference between facial paralysis and Palsy is cause for the paralysis can be identified, be it a tumor, infection, or nerve damage. Facial paralysis, in most cases, also appears more permanent than Bell's Palsy, with cases lasting for years to life if a patient doesn't seek treatment. Complete loss of ability to move facial muscles innervated by the facial nerve (i.e., the seventh cranial nerve)[1]

续 表

英文术语（中文术语）	定义（英文和/或中文）
Faciobranchial paresis(面臂轻瘫)	This pattern of paresis is highly suggestive of damage to the motor cortex, due to involvement of the superficial branches of the middle cerebral artery, but it is often seen in lesions involving the complete territory of the middle cerebral artery, the complete territory of the lenticulostriate arteries or the territory of the lateral lenticulostriate arteries. More rarely it was reported after anterior cerebral artery or brainstem infarcts[1]
Factor V Leiden Measurement(因子 V leidon 突变检测)	The determination of the amount of Factor V Leiden present in a sample[1]
Familial Combined Hyperlipidemias(家族性高胆固醇血症)	A type of familial lipid metabolism disorder characterized by a variable pattern of elevated plasma CHOLESTEROL and/or TRIGLYCERIDES. Multiple genes on different chromosomes may be involved, such as the major late transcription factor (UPSTREAM STIMULATORY FACTORS) on CHROMOSOME 1[1]
Fatty acid binding protein(脂肪酸结合蛋白质)	Fatty acid-binding proteins (FABPs) are a class of intracellular molecules involved in buffering and transporting long-chain fatty acids[1]
Fiber intake(纤维摄入)	fibre intake has been shown to have an inverse association with the risk of both haemorrhagic and ischaemic stroke[1]
Fibrinopeptide A(血纤维蛋白肽A)	Two small peptide chains removed from the N-terminal segment of the alpha chains of fibrinogen by the action of thrombin during the blood coagulation process. Each peptide chain contains 18 amino acid residues. In vivo, fibrinopeptide A is used as a marker to determine the rate of conversion of fibrinogen to fibrin by thrombin[1]
Fibromuscular dysplasia(肌纤维发育不良)	Fibromuscular dysplasia (FMD) is a non-atherosclerotic, non-inflammatory disease of the blood vessels that causes abnormal growth within the wall of an artery. FMD has been found in nearly every arterial bed in the body. However, the most common arteries affected are the renal and carotid arteries[1]
finger skin temperature biofeedback therapy(手指温度生物反馈疗法)	通过手指皮肤温度信号反馈进行治疗的方法。用于周围血液循环障碍、多发性神经炎等[3]

英文术语（中文术语）	定义（英文和/或中文）
Fish intake(鱼)	Fish consumption may be inversely associated with ischemic stroke but not with hemorrhagic stroke because of the potential antipla-telet aggregation property of LCn3PUFAs[1]
FLAIR weighted images(FLAIR加权图像)	A magnetic resonance imaging (MRI) pulse sequence that uses an inversion recovery technique to null fluids present in the imaging area, improving clarity of the object of interest[1]
Focal dystonia(局限性肌张力障碍)	A type of "dystonia" (HP:0001332) that is localized to a specific part of the body[2]
Focal dystonia(局限性肌张力障碍)	"肌张力障碍"（HP:0001332）的一种类型，局限于身体的特定部分[2]
Folic acid intake(叶酸摄入)	There is a positive correlation between homocysteine levels and stroke. For this reason, guidelines on the primary prevention of stroke recommend the use of folic acid in patients with known elevated homocysteine levels[1]
Forced grasping reflex(握持反射)	The grasp reflex is a flexion–adduction response in one or more digits, provoked by a distally moving pressure contact on a particular area of the palmar aspect of the hand[1]
Foville syndrome(Foville综合征)	Inferior medial pontine syndrome (or Foville syndrome) is one of the brainstem stroke syndromes occuring when there is infarction of the medial inferior aspect of the pons due to occlusion of the paramedian branches of the basilar artery. This infarction involves the following: - corticospinal tract leads to contralateral hemiplegia/hemiparesis. -corticobulbar tract leads to contralateral weakness of the lower half of the face. -medial leminiscus leads to contralateral loss of proprioception and vibration. -middle cerebellar peduncle leads to ipsilateral ataxia. -abducent nerve roots leads to lateral gaze paralysis and diplopia[1]

续　表

英文术语（中文术语）	定义（英文和/或中文）
Free radical synthesis(自由基合成)	free radical is an especially reactive atom or group of atoms that has one or more unpaired electrons; especially : one that is produced in the body by natural biological processes or introduced from outside (as in tobacco smoke, toxins, or pollutants) and that can damage cells, proteins, and DNA by altering their chemical structure. Free radicals cause lipid peroxidation, membrane damage, dysregulation of cellular processes, and mutations of the genome. In fact, reactive oxygen species can damage virtually any cellular component. Cell damage causes aberrations in ion homeostasis, cell signaling, and gene expression[1]
Frenchay Activities Index(Frenchay活动量表)	The Frenchay Activities Index is a useful stroke-specific instrument to assess functional status. Completion of the questionnaire is easy and takes only a few minutes. The Frenchay Activities Index has been developed specifically for measuring disability and handicap in stroke patients[1]
Frenchay Aphasia Screening Test(Frenchay构音障碍评价法)	The Frenchay Aphasia Screening Test is a reliable test which can be used by non-specialists to discriminate between aphasia and normal language[1]
Fruit(水果)	The fleshy or dry ripened ovary of a plant, enclosing the seed or seeds[1]
Fugl Meyer Assessment(Fugl-Meyer评定法)	One of the most widely recognized and clinically relevant measures of body function impairment after stroke is the Fugl-Meyer (FM) assessment. Of its 5 domains (motor, sensory, balance, range of motion, joint pain), the motor domain, which includes an assessment of the upper extremity (UE) and lower extremity (LE), has well-established reliability and validity as an indicator of motor impairment severity across different stroke recovery time points. Consistently, greater motor severity as indicated by lower UE and LE FM motor scores is correlated with lower functional ability, such as spontaneous arm use for feeding, dressing and grooming,6 or walking at functional gait speeds[1]
Functional Ambulation Category(功能性步行量表)	The FAC has excellent reliability, good concurrent and predictive validity, and good responsiveness in patients with hemiparesis after stroke[1]

英文术语（中文术语）	定义（英文和/或中文）
Functional Ambulation Category(功能性步行量表)	The Functional Ambulation Classification (FAC) was an early method for classifying mobility. The primary aim in the development of the FAC was to establish a clinically meaningful outcome measure of mobility. Secondary aims were to devise an inexpensive measure that required little time for therapist training and administration, yet was reliable and valid[1]
Functional comorbidity index(功能性共病指数)	The FCI was developed as a comorbidity index with physical function as the outcome of interest, using an 18-item (comorbidities) self-administered questionnaire where the FCI score is the sum of the number of conditions reported for the person (0–18)[1]
functional electrical stimulation therapy(功能性电刺激疗法)	用低频脉冲电流按照预先设计的程序刺激已丧失功能的器官或肢体，以所产生的即时效应来代替或纠正器官或肢体功能进行日常活动的康复治疗。如：功能性行走、排尿、排便、吞咽等功能控制[3]
Furosemide(呋塞米)	Loop diuretics like furosemide may act by decreasing total body water and increasing blood osmolality, thereby removing water from the brain[1]
Gait apraxia(步态失用)	Gait apraxia affecting the ability to make walking movements with the legs[2]
Gait apraxia(步态失用)	步态失用指指挥腿行走的能力受损[2]
Gait ataxia(共济失调步态)	A type of "ataxia" (HP:0001251) characterized by the impairment of the ability to coordinate the movements required for normal walking[2]
Gait ataxia(共济失调步态)	"共济失调"(HP:0001251)的一种类型，表现为正常行走时所需的协同运动能力受损[2]
galvanic skin response biofeedback therapy(直流电皮肤反应生物反馈疗法)	通过皮肤电阻信号反馈进行治疗的方法。用于自主神经功能紊乱等[3]
Gastritis(胃炎)	Inflammation of the GASTRIC MUCOSA, a lesion observed in a number of unrelated disorders[1]
Gaze-evoked horizontal nystagmus(凝视诱发性水平眼震)	Horizontal nystagmus made apparent by looking to the right or to the left[2]
Gaze-evoked horizontal nystagmus(凝视诱发性水平眼震)	水平性眼球震颤在看向右侧或左侧时变得明显[2]

续 表

英文术语（中文术语）	定义（英文和/或中文）
Gaze-evoked nystagmus(凝视诱发性眼球震颤)	Nystagmus made apparent by looking to the right or to the left [2]
Gaze-evoked nystagmus(凝视诱发性眼球震颤)	眼球震颤在向右或向左凝视的时候变得明显 [2]
Gene expression(基因表达)	Transient focal cerebral ischemia induces a complex change in genomic profile, including expression of new genes, upregulation and downregulation of genes, occurring distinctly in a temporal manner. Detection of gene changes after ischemia is just the first step towards understanding different molecular pathways and proteomics and peptidomics studies provides supplemental insights [1]
Generalized dystonia(全身型肌张力障碍)	A type of "dystonia" (HP:0001332) that affects all or most of the body [2]
Generalized dystonia(全身型肌张力障碍)	"肌张力障碍"(HP:0001332)的一种类型，累及所有或大部分的身体 [2]
Gerstmann syndrome(Gerstmann综合征)	Gerstmann syndrome, also known as angular gyrus syndrome, is a dominant hemisphere stroke syndrome consisting of four components: agraphia or dysgraphia acalculia or dyscalculia finger agnosia left-right disorientation Pure Gerstmann syndrome is said to be without aphasia [1]
Glaucomatous visual field defect(青光眼性视野缺损)	Glaucomatous visual field defect [2]
Glaucomatous visual field defect(青光眼性视野缺损)	青光眼造成的视野缺损 [2]
Glial fibrillary acidic protein(胶质纤维酸性蛋白)	Glial fibrillary-associated protein (GFAP) is a monomeric intermediate filament protein present in astrocytes and, to a lesser degree, in ependymal cells of the brain, where it functions as a part of the cytoskeleton. GFAP is a brain-specific intermediate filament protein found in astrocytes. It was identified as a candidate biomarker ICH in the acute phase [1]
Glutathione(谷胱甘肽)	A tripeptide with many roles in cells. It conjugates to drugs to make them more soluble for excretion, is a cofactor for some enzymes, is involved in protein disulfide bond rearrangement and reduces peroxides [1]

续 表

英文术语（中文术语）	定义（英文和/或中文）
Glutathione S transferase P(谷胱甘肽 S 转移酶 P)	a molecule involved in detoxifying ROS[1]
Glutathione S transferase P(谷胱甘肽 S 转移酶 P)	A transferase that catalyzes the addition of aliphatic, aromatic, or heterocyclic FREE RADICALS as well as EPOXIDES and arene oxides to GLUTATHIONE. Addition takes place at the SULFUR. It also catalyzes the reduction of polyol nitrate by glutathione to polyol and nitrite[1]
Glycerol(甘油)	The sugar glycerol is another osmotic agent that may also has neuroprotective properties. In human stroke, increase of blood flow to ischemic territories and improvement in ischemic brain energy metabolism after glycerol administration have also been postulated[1]
Grain(谷物)	Whole-grain intake was associated with a trend towards a reduction in the incidence of stroke[1]
Graphomania(书写狂)	Graphomania, also known as scribomania, refers to an obsessive impulse to write[1]
group language training(小组语言训练)	把失语症患者编成小组，形成日常交流的真实情景，进行语言训练的一种方法。目的是通过相互接触，学会将个人训练的成果，在实际中有效地应用[3]
Guiding airflow method(引导气流法)	引导气流通过口腔，减少鼻漏气的训练方法。如吹吸管、吹乒乓球、吹喇叭、吹哨子、吹奏乐器、吹蜡烛、吹羽毛、吹纸张，都可以用来集中和引导气流[3]
Hallucinations(幻觉)	a sensory perception in the absence of an external stimulus. Hallucinations are often differentiated from sensory illusions which are distortions or misinterpretations of actual sensory experiences. Hallucinations can involve any sensory modality (visual, auditory, tactile, olfactory, or gustatory). Simple (unformed) hallucinations are sensory perceptions that are typically vague and without meaning (e.g., whistling sounds, flashing lights, geometric patterns)[1]
Hallucinations(幻觉)	Perceptions in a conscious and awake state in the absence of external stimuli which have qualities of real perception, in that they are vivid, substantial, and located in external objective space[2]

续 表

英文术语（中文术语）	定义（英文和/或中文）
Hallucinations(幻觉)	在有意识的、清醒状态下，缺乏真实的外界刺激的一种感觉，因此他们是生动的、实质性的、并存在于外部客观空间[2]
Haptoglobin(结合珠蛋白)	Haptoglobin is a major acute-phase proteins (APP) in numerous species whose synthesis is increased several-fold by inflammation or injury, and has proven useful in the diagnosis of tissue injury and infectious disease[1]
Head tremor(头部震颤)	An unintentional, oscillating to-and-fro muscle movement affecting head movement[2]
Head tremor(头部震颤)	无意识的，影响头部运动的反复的肌肉振荡运动[2]
Headache(头痛)	A headache is a pain or discomfort that is perceived to be in the head, although sometimes the pain may actually be referred from other structures such as the neck. Lifethreatening causes of headache, although rare, must be considered as more expedient treatment can be life saving[1]
heart rate bio-feedback therapy(心率生物反馈疗法)	通过心率信号反馈进行治疗的方法。心率反馈可以控制多种不同的心律紊乱。治疗时，患者的心率被监视，并告知患者心率的变化和波动。用于神经症、心律不齐、心动过速等[3]
Heart type fatty acid binding protein(心脏型脂肪酸结合蛋白)	H-FABP is present in multiple tissue types and has found application as a biomarker for acute myocardial infarction[1]
heat therapy(热疗法)	以各种热源为介质，将热直接作用于人体治疗疾病的方法[3]
heavy drinking(酗酒)	Drinking an excessive amount of ALCOHOLIC BEVERAGES in a short period of time[1]
Hematologic Tests(血液检测)	Tests used in the analysis of the hemic system[1]
Hemianacusia(单侧聋)	Hemianacusia means the loss of hearing in one ear. Unilateral cortical temporal strokes produce subtle hearing dysfunction. Pure-tone thresholds and speech discrimination remain largely preserved; dysfunction becomes apparent in tests with distorted and dichotic stimuli. Unilateral cortical lesions produce contralateral ear extinction. Sound localization is impaired in the sound field contralateral to the impaired temporal lobe and also in the vertical plane. There exist, in addition, differences between right and left lesions[1]

英文术语（中文术语）	定义（英文和/或中文）
Hemianopia(偏盲)	A binocular visual defect in each eye's hemifield. Hemianopia is due to infarction of the striate visual cortex on the banks of the calcarine fissure, a region supplied by the calcarine branch of the PCA, or is explained by interruption of the geniculocalcarine tract as it nears the visual cortex [1]
Hemianopia(偏盲)	Partial or complete loss of vision in one half of the visual field of one or both eyes [2]
Hemianopia(偏盲)	一只或两只眼睛的半侧视野局部或全部的丧失 [2]
Hemiataxia(偏身共济失调)	Hemiataxia is a common occurrence in thalamic infarction involving the ventrolateral part of the thalamus usually from involvement of the thalamogeniculate territory [1]
Hemiballismus(单侧抽搐)	Hemiballism is a rare hyperkinetic movement disorder, characterized by irregular, wide amplitude and vigorous involuntary movements of the unilateral limbs. The term ballismus is derived from the Greek word meaning "to throw" because the abnormal movements resemble the motions of throwing. The movements are usually continuous but may be intermittent and can be voluntarily restrained by the patient, although only for a few minutes. They are most prominent during periods of rest but are absent during sleep. It may occur with other types of involuntary movements, such as dystonia, myoclonus, or orofacial gestures. Hemiballism is often used interchangeably but distinguished from hemichorea by the fact that hemichoreic movements are slower, more randomly distributed, less violent, and primarily involve distal musculature. Some patients with hemiballism also have choreiform movements; therefore, the bhemiballism-hemichoreaQ is often used to describe this clinical spectrum [1]
Hemifacial spasm(偏侧面肌痉挛)	A segmental myoclonus of muscles innervated by the facial nerve [2]
Hemifacial spasm(偏侧面肌痉挛)	面神经支配肌肉的节段性肌阵挛 [2]
Hemihypesthesia(偏身感觉减退)	Diminished sensibility in one side of the body [1]

续　表

英文术语（中文术语）	定义（英文和/或中文）
hemihypoesthesia without cognitive impairment(无认知障碍的偏身感觉减退)	Diminished sensibility in one side of the body. A rarer but typical presentation of AChA infarcts is the triad of contralateral severe hemiparesis, hemihypesthesia and upper quadrantanopsia or contralateral versus ipsilateral hemianopsia (in the case of lateral geniculate body or optic tract, respectively) without cognitive disturbances, in contrast with MCA infarction[1]
Hemihypokinesia(少动症)	Hemihypokinesia is found in right hemispheric strokes as part of motor hemineglect, but can be found in basal ganglia strokes, including the thalamus, and catatonia in biparietal infarcts[1]
Hemimedullary infarction symptom(延髓半侧综合征)	The hemimedullary syndrome is very rare and includes Wallenberg's presentation with Déjerine's syndrome, leading to contralateral motor and allmodalities sensory deficits, ipsilateral tongue, pharynx and vocal cord weakness and facial thermoalgesic deficit, ipsilateral ataxia and Horner's syndrome[1]
Hemineglect(偏侧忽略)	Hemispatial neglect is one element of the neglect syndrome. Neglect is operationally defined as the failure to report, respond or orient either to external sensory stimulation or mental representations of sensory events when the failure is not attributable to a primary sensory or motor deficit[1]
Hemiparesis(轻偏瘫)	Loss of strength in the arm, leg, and sometimes face on one side of the body. Hemiplegia refers to a complete loss of strength, whereas hemiparesis refers to an incomplete loss of strength[1]
Hemispheric Stroke Scale(半球卒中量表)	The Hemispheric Stroke Scale is a 100-point neurologic assessment scale. This comprehensive scale measures level of consciousness, language, cortical function, motor function, and sensory capacity, with higher scores reflecting more deficits[1]
Heparin(肝素)	heparin has been used to treat thrombosis and stroke. Its anticoagulant action may retard the advance of cerebral thromboembolism while arterial recanalisation occurs and, by preventing deep venous thrombosis, it may decrease the incidence of pulmonary embolism - one of the causes of death following stroke[1]

英文术语（中文术语）	定义（英文和/或中文）
Hereditary hemorrhagic telangiectasia(遗传性出血性毛细血管扩张症)	An autosomal dominant disease characterized by the presence of multiple arteriovenous malformations that lack intervening capillaries and result in direct connections between arteries and veins[1]
Heroin(海洛因)	Heroin is an opioid painkiller and the 3,6-diacetyl ester of morphine. Heroin is prescribed as an analgesic, cough suppressant and as an antidiarrhoeal[1]
Heteronymous hemianopia(对侧偏盲)	Heteronymous hemianopia[2]
Heteronymous hemianopia(对侧偏盲)	双眼不同侧视力障碍[2]
Hiccups(呃逆)	Hiccup may be regarded as a failure of the usual alternative excitation–inhibition between glottis closure and inspiration. The coordinating centre is located in the brainstem reticular formation. Hiccup is one of the typical transient symptoms appearing at the onset of a lateral medullary stroke; it may become chronic[1]
High alpha linolenic acid intake(高α-亚麻酸摄入量)	low intakes of alpha-linolenic acid may be a risk factor for stroke[1]
High intracranial pressure(颅内压增高)	Intracranial pressure (ICP) is the pressure that is exerted on the brain, cerebrospinal fluid, and blood within the skull. In an adult at rest, it is usually less than 10–15mm of Mercury. If ICP rises above normal due to trauma, hydrocephalus, hemorrhage, or tumor, patients can exhibit behavioral changes, headache, decreased consciousness, somnolence, lethargy, seizures, and/or vomiting[1]
High magnesium intake(高镁摄入量)	Magnesium intake is, like potassium intake, inversely associated with the risk of stroke, ischaemic stroke in particular[1]
High potassium intake(高钾饮食)	higher level of potassium intake has been associated with a reduced risk of stroke in prospective studies. The recommended potassium intake >4.7 g/d (120 mmol/d)[1]
Histological biomarkers of stroke(脑卒中的组织学生物标志物)	Histological markers can be especially useful in evaluating uncommon causes, such as vasculitis and collagen vascular diseases[1]
Homonymous hemianopia(同向性偏盲)	Homonymous hemianopia[2]

续　表

英文术语（中文术语）	定义（英文和/或中文）
Homonymous hemianopia(同向性偏盲)	Homonymous hemianopia is a visual field defect involving either the two right or the two left halves of the visual fields of both eyes. Homonymous hemianopia is usually congruent and complete, sometimes sparing part of the upper quadrant[1]
Homonymous hemianopia(同向性偏盲)	双眼同侧视力障碍[2]
Homonymous quadrantanopsia(同侧象限盲)	Homonymous quadrantanopsia is defined as the visual loss that is restricted to one quadrant of the visual field and is comparable in both eyes. Thus, when looking straight ahead, patients may have difficulty seeing objects or movement in the upper or lower quadrant of the visual field, but it will be in the same quadrant (i.e., either to the right or to the left) regardless of which eye is being tested. Depending on the extent of the lesion, slightlymore or slightly less than one quarter of the visual field may actually be affected. Homonymous quadrantanopsia usually results from lesions posterior to the lateral geniculate nuclei, which encroach either on the optic radiations or the primary visual cortex[1]
Horizontal conjugate gaze palsy(水平共轭注视麻痹)	Conjugate-gaze palsy is one of the most common eyemovement abnormalities in patients with acute stroke. The eyes may be deviated to one side, either to the side of a hemispheral lesion or to the opposite side of a pons lesion, with gaze paresis towards the opposite side[1]
Horizontal gaze paresis(水平凝视麻痹)	Lateral gaze palsy is an inability to produce horizontal, conjugate eye movements in one or both directions. Lesions of the cranial nerve VI (abducens) nucleus in the pons cause ipsilateral, horizontal gaze palsy by disrupting motoneurons that innervate the ipsilateral lateral rectus muscle by way of cranial nerve VI, and interneurons that connect to the contralateral cranial nerve III nucleus in the midbrain, via the medial longitudinal fasciculus, to stimulate the medial rectus of the opposite eye. Lesions of the paramedian pontine reticular formation, adjacent to the abducens nucleus, may cause lateral gaze palsy, particularly involving ipsilateral saccadic eye movements. Lesions of the frontal or parietal cortical eye fields may also cause weakness of horizontal gaze (contralateral to frontal lesions and ipsilateral to parietal lesions) that becomes more subtle over time[1]

英文术语（中文术语）	定义（英文和/或中文）
Horizontal ipsilateral gaze palsy(水平同侧注视麻痹)	Horizontal-gaze abnormalities are more common than vertical ones. Because the horizontal-gaze system depends on unilateral gaze centers and pathways, it is more vulnerable than the vertical-gaze system, which has bilateral input. Horizontal-gaze paresis can vary from (a) gaze-evoked nystagmus to (b) slowing or dysmetria of the movement to (c) a total inability to move the eyes in the involved direction of gaze. Severe gaze paralysis results in conjugate deviation of the eyes in the opposite direction at rest. The most common abnormalities in this group are gaze palsies resulting from a cerebrovascular accident (CVA). Localization of the lesion depends on concurrent neurologic findings such as hemiparesis, visual field loss, and cranial nerve palsies. The following discussion covers saccade abnormalities first and then pursuit abnormalities. An isolated horizontal-gaze paresis is rare. The lesion can be located anywhere in the horizontal-gaze pathways and cannot be localized more specifically without other neurologic signs and symptoms[1]
Horizontal ipsilateral gaze palsy(水平同侧注视麻痹)	Lesions that involve the abducens nucleus produce ipsilateral horizontal gaze palsy. The abducens nucleus lies in close proximity to the horizontal gaze center and facial nerve genu within the lower pons at the floor of the fourth ventricle[1]
Horizontal jerk nystagmus(水平跳动性眼球震颤)	Nystagmus consisting of horizontal to-and-fro eye movements, in which the movement in one direction is faster than in the other[2]
Horizontal jerk nystagmus(水平跳动性眼球震颤)	眼球震颤包括水平至往复眼球运动，在其中一个方向上的运动比在其它方向上更快[2]
Horizontal nystagmus(水平性眼震)	Nystagmus consisting of horizontal to-and-fro eye movements[2]
Horizontal nystagmus(水平性眼震)	眼球震颤由横向来回的眼球运动组成[2]
horizontal optokinetic nystagmus(水平性视动性眼球震颤)	Horizontal opticokinetic nystagmus[2]
horizontal optokinetic nystagmus(水平性视动性眼球震颤)	水平性视动性的眼球震颤[2]

续　表

英文术语（中文术语）	定义（英文和/或中文）
Horizontal pendular nystagmus(水平钟摆性眼球震颤)	Nystagmus consisting of horizontal to-and-fro eye movements of equal velocity[2]
Horizontal pendular nystagmus(水平钟摆性眼球震颤)	由横向往复的等速眼球运动组成的眼球震颤[2]
Horner syndrome(霍纳综合征)	An abnormality resulting from a lesion of the sympathetic nervous system characterized by a combination of unilateral ptosis, miosis, and often ipsilateral hypohidrosis and conjunctival injection[2]
Horner syndrome(霍纳综合征)	Ptosis, miosis, and occasionally apparent enophthalmos and anhidrosis on one side of the face, loss of ciliospinal reflex and blood shot conjunctiva. An abnormality resulting from a lesion of the sympathetic nervous system characterized by a combination of unilateral ptosis, miosis, and often ipsilateral hypohidrosis and conjunctival injection[1]
Horner syndrome(霍纳综合征)	异常特征由交感神经系统的损伤而引起，表现为单方面上睑下垂、瞳孔缩小，并经常同侧少汗和结膜下注射[2]
Hufschmidt therapy(痉挛肌电刺激疗法)	应用低频电刺激痉挛肌和/或拮抗肌以缓解肌肉痉挛为主要目的的治疗方法。常用频率为0.66～1Hz，波宽为0.2～0.5ms的单路或双路方波电流，双路电流交替刺激时的刺激时间差常为0.1～1.5s[3]
Hydroxyl radicals(羟基自由基)	hydroxyl radical is the most reactive free radical which plays an important role in tissue damage caused by radiation. the hydroxyl radical (OH) causes DNA fragmentation. OH is also known to induce lipid peroxidation of fatty acid side chains of membrance phospholipids[1]
Hypercholesteremia(高胆固醇血症)	A condition with abnormally high levels of CHOLESTEROL in the blood. It is defined as a cholesterol value exceeding the 95th percentile for the population[1]
Hyperglycemia(高血糖)	Hyperglycemia is common in patients with acute stroke, occurring in up to 60% of patients overall and approximately 12- 53% of acute stroke patients without a prior diagnosis of diabetes. Hyperglycaemia predicts higher mortality and morbidity after acute stroke independently of other adverse prognostic factors, such as older age, type and severity of stroke, and non-reversibility of the neurological deficit[1]

英文术语（中文术语）	定义（英文和/或中文）
Hypergraphia(强迫书写)	Hypergraphia is a behavioral condition characterized by the intense desire to write [1]
Hyperlipidaemia(高脂血症)	Conditions with excess LIPIDS in the blood. Abnormally high level of lipids in blood [1]
Hyperlipoproteinemias(高脂蛋白血症)	Conditions with abnormally elevated levels of LIPOPROTEINS in the blood. They may be inherited, acquired, primary, or secondary. Hyperlipoproteinemias are classified according to the pattern of lipoproteins on electrophoresis or ultracentrifugation [1]
Hypersomnia(嗜睡)	Poststroke hypersomnia can be defined on clinical grounds as an exaggerated sleep propensity with excessive daytime sleepiness, increased daytime napping, or prolonged nighttime sleep following cerebrovascular event. As a consequence, patients may be difficult to arouse or keep awake once awakened [1]
Hypertension(高血压)	Hypertension is usually defined by the presence of a chronic elevation of systemic arterial pressure above a certain threshold value [1]
Hypertonic Saline(高渗盐水)	Over the past few years, hypertonic saline solutions have increasingly been used as an alternative to mannitol to control brain edema of various types. As is the case with mannitol, several mechanisms may be responsible for the reduction of brain edema achieved with hypertonic saline. Because sodium chloride is completely excluded from an intact BBB, it has been proposed that hypertonic saline may be a more favorable osmotic agent compared with mannitol. Furthermore, hypertonic saline has the effect of expanding the intravascular volume with increasing mean arterial blood pressure leading to improved CPP, whereas mannitol is an osmotic diuretic that secondary leads to volume depletion. Other proposed mechanisms of action include modulation of inflammatory response and neuron excitation, and improved oxygenation [1]
Hypertriglyceridemia(高甘油三酯血症)	A condition of elevated levels of TRIGLYCERIDES in the blood [1]

续　表

英文术语（中文术语）	定义（英文和/或中文）
Hyperventilation(过度换气)	Hyperventilation is one of the most effective methods available for the rapid reduction of ICP. The CO2 reactivity of intracerebral vessels is one of the normal mechanisms involved in the regulation of CBF[1]
Hypervigilance(过度警觉)	Hypervigilance may be caused by an increase in activity of systems maintaining wakefulness or by impairment of sleep promoting mechanisms as can occur with lesions of the anterior hypothalamus, thalamus or brainstem. Hypervigilance, insomnia, inversion of sleep–wake cycle and delirium often coexist in the same patient[1]
Hypnic headache(睡眠性头痛)	A headache disorder that occurs exclusively at night, waking the affected individual from sleep[2]
Hypnic headache(睡眠性头痛)	仅仅发生在夜间的头痛，可导致患者痛醒[2]
Hypoglycemia(低血糖)	Hypoglycemia is characterized by extremely low blood glucose levels. Although 60–70 mg/dL (or milligrams per deciliter) is typically cited as the lower level for normal glucose, different values have also been proposed. Hypoglycemia is commonly associated with, among other symptoms, generalized discomfort, sweating, weakness, irritability, tremor, and poor motor coordination[1]
Hypoglycemic coma(低血糖昏迷)	Coma caused by low blood sugar, when venous plasma glucose concentration below 2.8mmol / L[2]
Hypoglycemic coma(低血糖昏迷)	由低血糖导致的昏迷，静脉血浆葡萄糖浓度低于2.8mmol/L可引起[2]
Hypophonia(发音过弱)	Hypophonia has been defined as a reduction in speech volume. It is an uncommon finding in acute stroke, mainly related to multiple deep infarcts[1]
Hypotension(低血压)	Occurs when blood pressure is reduced to <= 90/60 mmHg[1]
Hypothermia(低体温)	Hypothermia reduces the cerebral metabolic rate, stabilizes BBB, reduces brain edema, free radical formation, and the release of excitatory neurotransmitters, and attenuates postischemic inflammatory response and apoptosis[1]

英文术语（中文术语）	定义（英文和/或中文）
Ideomotor apraxia(观念运动性失用)	Patients with ideomotor apraxia fail to execute purposeful, skilled or learned movements without this being due to elementary sensorimotor, extrapyramidal, or other cognitive disturbances. The disorder affects both the limbs contralateral and ipsilateral to a unilateral lesion which practically always involves the left hemisphere (in right handed subjects) [1]
Immune responce(免疫应答)	The immune response to acute cerebral ischemia is a major factor in stroke pathobiology and outcome. While the immune response starts locally in occluded and hypoperfused vessels and the ischemic brain parenchyma, inflammatory mediators generated in situ propagate through the organism as a whole [1]
Impulsivity(冲动)	Impulsivity is defined as a personality trait characterized by the inclination of an individual to initiate behavior without adequate forethought as to the consequences of his or her actions (impulse action), thus acting on the spur of the moment [1]
Indomethacin(吲哚美辛)	Indomethacin is a potent cerebral vasoconstrictor that also may exhibit antiedema and anti-inflammatory effects. ICP-lowering capacity of indomethacin has been described in few case reports on head trauma [1]
Inducible nitric oxide synthase(诱导型一氧化氮合酶)	Inducible nitric oxide synthase (iNOS) is a key enzyme in the macrophage inflammatory response, which is the source of nitric oxide (NO) that is potently induced in response to proinflammatory stimuli [1]
Inflammatory disorder(炎性疾病)	Inflammatory abnormalities are a large group of disorders that underlie a vast variety of human diseases. The immune system is often involved with inflammatory disorders, demonstrated in both allergic reactions and some myopathies, with many immune system disorders resulting in abnormal inflammation. Non-immune diseases with etiological origins in inflammatory processes include cancer, atherosclerosis, and ischaemic heart disease [1]

续　表

英文术语（中文术语）	定义（英文和/或中文）
Inflammatory response(炎症)	Ischemic injury triggers inflammatory cascades in the brain parenchyma that may further amplify tissue damage by many mechanisms. Within minutes of occlusion, there occurs upregulation of proinflammatory genes which produces mediators of inflammation such as platelet-activating factor, tumor necrosis factor α, and interleukin 1 β[1]
Insomnia(失眠)	Difficulty with sleep initiation or maintenance or unintended early awakenings. Insomnia is defined by difficulty initiating or maintaining sleep, early awakenings, insufficient sleep quality, and corresponding poor daytime functioning (lack of energy, fatigue, concentration problems, mood swings, irritability). Particularly in patients with subcortical, thalamic, thalamomesencephalic, and large tegmental pontine stroke, insomnia may be accompanied by an inversion of the sleep-wake cycle with insomnia and agitation during the night and hypersomnia during the day[1]
Insulin resistance(胰岛素抵抗)	Diminished effectiveness of INSULIN in lowering blood sugar levels: requiring the use of 200 units or more of insulin per day to prevent HYPERGLYCEMIA or KETOSIS[1]
Intention tremor(意向性震颤)	An oscillatory cerebellar ataxia that tends to be absent when the limbs are inactive and during the first part of voluntary movement but worsening as the movement continues and greater precision is required (e.g., in touching a target such as the patient's nose or a physician's finger)[2]
Intention tremor(意向性震颤)	摆动性小脑性共济失调，肢体静止或刚开始随意运动时消失，持续运动和需要更加精准时加重（例如，触摸目标如患者的鼻子或医生的手指）[2]
Inter-α-trypsin inhibitor heavy chain H3(胰蛋白酶抑制剂重链H3)	A protein that is a translation product of the human ITIH3 gene[1]
Intercellular Adhesion Molecule 1(细胞间黏附分子1)	A cell-surface ligand involved in leukocyte adhesion and inflammation. Its production is induced by gamma-interferon and it is required for neutrophil migration into inflamed tissue[1]

续　表

英文术语（中文术语）	定义（英文和/或中文）
Interleukin 1(白细胞介素-1)	A soluble factor produced by MONOCYTES; MACROPHAGES, and other cells which activates T-lymphocytes and potentiates their response to mitogens or antigens. Interleukin-1 is a general term refers to either of the two distinct proteins, INTERLEUKIN-1ALPHA and INTERLEUKIN-1BETA. The biological effects of IL-1 include the ability to replace macrophage requirements for T-cell activation [1]
Interleukin 10(白细胞介素-10)	IL-10 is a major anti-inflammatory molecule in various organ injuries. It is produced by infiltrating immune cells and reactive glial cells after ischemic brain injury. Viral overexpression of IL-10 in ischemic brain is neuroprotective [1]
Interleukin 23(白细胞介素-23)	IL-23 and IL-1β activate T cell-mediated innate immunity and promote secondary ischemic damage during the subacute phase of ischemic brain injury [1]
Interleukin 6(白细胞介素-6)	A cytokine that stimulates the growth and differentiation of B-LYMPHOCYTES and is also a growth factor for HYBRIDOMAS and plasmacytomas. It is produced by many different cells including T-LYMPHOCYTES; MONOCYTES; and FIBROBLASTS [1]
Internal carotid artery dissection(颈内动脉夹层)	Internal carotid artery dissection is kind of cervical artery dissection [1]
Internal carotid artery infarction syndrome (颈内动脉梗死综合征)	Embolic occlusion of the ICA, either proximally or distally, usually leads to severe stroke, showing concomitant signs of all anterior circulation arteries. A progressive atherosclerotic occlusion is usually less severe, with a classic subacute two-phase presentation or even asymptomatic. Retinal ischemia from carotid emboli may be transient (amaurosis fugax) or persistent [1]
intonation training(语调训练)	改变患者说话时音调低或单一音调的训练方法。训练时要指出患者的音调问题，训练者可以发音由低到高，让患者模仿，也可以利用乐器让患者随音阶变化发声来克服音调单一问题。另外，也可以用可视言语训练仪器进行辅助训练 [3]

续　表

英文术语（中文术语）	定义（英文和/或中文）
Intra-arterial thrombolysis(血管内溶栓)	Intra-arterial therapy (IAT) for acute ischemic stroke refers to endovascular catheter-based approaches to achieve recanalization using mechanical clot disruption, locally injected thrombolytic agents or both. IAT may be used in addition to intravenous tissue plasminogen activator (tPA) or in patients who do not qualify for tPA, usually because they are outside the approved 3-h timeframe window or have contraindications, such as elevated international normalized ratio or partial thromboplastin time[1]
Intravenous Recombinant Tissue Plasminogen Activator(静脉重组组织纤溶酶原激活剂)	Intravenous administration of rtPA is the only FDA-approved medical therapy for treatment of patients with acute ischemic stroke[1]
Intravenous thrombolysis(静脉溶栓)	Intravenous (IV) thrombolysis with tissue plasminogen activator (tPA, alteplase) is the standard of care in the treatment of acute ischemic stroke in current clinical practice and the extension of the time window up to 4.5 hours after symptoms onset has been already approved by the European Medicines Agency (EMEA) and US Food and Drug Administration (FDA) agency and included in European and American guidelines recommendations[1]
Ipsilateral conjugate gaze palsy(同侧共轭注视麻痹)	Conjugate-gaze palsy is one of the most common eyemovement abnormalities in patients with acute stroke. The eyes may be deviated to one side, either to the side of a hemispheral lesion or to the opposite side of a pons lesion, with gaze paresis towards the opposite side[1]
Ipsilateral facial paralysis(同侧面瘫)	Facial paralysis can be caused by compression of the facial nerve.The main difference between facial paralysis and Palsy is cause for the paralysis can be identified, be it a tumor, infection, or nerve damage. Facial paralysis, in most cases, also appears more permanent than Bell's Palsy, with cases lasting for years to life if a patient doesn't seek treatment. Complete loss of ability to move facial muscles innervated by the facial nerve (i.e., the seventh cranial nerve)[1]

英文术语（中文术语）	定义（英文和/或中文）
Ipsilateral gait ataxia(同侧步态共济失调)	A type of ataxia characterized by the impairment of the ability to coordinate the movements required for normal walking. Gait ataxia is characeirzed by a wide-based staggering gait with a tendency to fall[1]
Ipsilateral hearing loss(同侧听力丧失)	Medical definitions of deafness refer to impairment in the physical structures necessary for hearing and understanding language. The term "deaf" refers to a degree of hearing loss that significantly impacts access to auditory language; "hard of hearing" typically refers to hearing loss that still allows for some access to auditory information[1]
Ipsilateral limb ataxia(同侧肢体共济失调)	A kind of ataxia that affects movements of the extremities. Limb ataxia is generally caused by lesions of the cerebellar hemispheres and associated pathways[1]
Ipsilateral nystagmus(同侧眼球震颤)	Rhythmic, involuntary oscillations of one or both eyes related to abnormality in fixation, conjugate gaze, or vestibular mechanisms[1]
Ipsilateral third cranial nerve palsy(同侧第三颅神经麻痹)	Damage to the oculomotor nerve (III) can cause double vision (diplopia) and inability to coordinate the movements of both eyes (strabismus), also eyelid drooping (ptosis) and pupil dilation (mydriasis)[1]
Ipsilateral third cranial nerve palsy(同侧第三颅神经麻痹)	Reduced ability to control the movement of the eye associated with damage to the third cranial nerve (the oculomotor nerve)[1]
Ipsilateral tongue paralysis(同侧舌肌麻痹)	Ipsilateral tongue paralysis is the least common but most topographically localizing sign of medial medullary infarction. Tongue weakness is probably most often related to involvement of the intraparenchymal XIIth nerve fibres as they pass ventrally to exit at the medullary base rather than to infarction of the hypoglossal nucleus in the tegmentum. Tongue paresis causes slurring of speech especially of lingual consonants[1]
IQ motif containing GTPase activation protein 1(含有 GTPase 激活蛋白1的IQ基序)	IQGAP1 is an evolutionarily conserved scaffold protein that plays a fundamental role in cell polarity[1]

续 表

英文术语（中文术语）	定义（英文和/或中文）
Ischemic modified albumin(缺血修饰白蛋白)	Albumin is the most abundant protein found in plasma, functioning as a nonspecific carrier molecule and maintaining oncotic pressure. In the context of ischemia, structural changes occur at the N-terminus of the protein, possibly as a result of exposure to ROS. This change in the albumin protein is detected by a cobalt-binding test. Over the last decade, increased ischemia-modified albumin concentration has been linked to acute myocardial ischemia, limb ischemia, mesenteric ischemia and deep venous thrombosis . Serum levels of ischemia-modified albumin are increased in subjects with both ischemic and hemorrhagic stroke compared with controls at baseline[1]
Isolated dysarthria(孤立性构音障碍)	Isolated dysarthria is an atypical lacunar syndrome and may represent a clinical manifestation of "dysarthria-clumsy hand syndrome."[1]
Isolated monoparesis(孤立单肢轻瘫)	Isolated monoparesis can be the clinical presentation in up to 4% of patients with lacunar infarcts[1]
Isometric tremor(等轴性震颤)	An isometric tremor occurs with muscle contraction against a rigid stationary object (e.g., when making a fist)[2]
Isometric tremor(等轴性震颤)	对于刚性静止物体（如拳头），肌肉收缩时发生等轴震颤[2]
Kinetic tremor(运动性震颤)	Tremor that occurs during any voluntary movement. It may include visually or non-visually guided movements. Tremor during target directed movement is called intention tremor[2]
Kinetic tremor(运动性震颤)	在任何随意运动中发生的震颤。它可以包括视觉或非视觉指导的运动。随意运动期间的震颤称为意图震颤[2]
Lack of spontaneity(自发性行为缺乏)	In language, verbal adynamia (lack of spontaneity of speech) is seen with lesions of the medial frontal lobes and refers to difficulty in initiation and maintenance of language output[1]
Lacunar stroke syndrome(腔隙性脑梗死症状)	Lacunar stroke syndrome (LACS) is a description of the clinical syndrome that results from a lacunar infarct[1]
Large central visual field defect(中心视野缺损较大)	Large central visual field defect[2]
Large vessel atherosclerosis(大动脉粥样硬化)	Large vessel atherosclerotic disease, most commonly extracranial carotid stenosis, accounts for some 15–20% of cerebral ischemic events[1]

英文术语（中文术语）	定义（英文和/或中文）
Laryngeal dystonia(喉部肌张力障碍)	A form of focal dystonia that affects the vocal cords, associated with involuntary contractions of the vocal cords causing interruptions of speech and affecting the voice quality and often leading to patterned, repeated breaks in speech [2]
Laryngeal dystonia(喉部肌张力障碍)	一种影响声带的局灶肌张力障碍类型，声带不自主的收缩导致言语中断，影响声音质量，常常导致模式化的反复言语中断 [2]
Limb apraxia(肢体失用)	Difficulty in performing the correct execution of limbs movements in absence of motor impairment [2]
Limb apraxia(肢体失用)	Limb-kinetic apraxia is the inability to make finely graded, precise limb movements. It has been difficult to separate this form of apraxia from motor dysfunction related to elemental motor disturbance, and it remains controversial that this is actually an apraxic disorder of learned skilled movement [1]
Limb apraxia(肢体失用)	在没有运动障碍的情况下难以正确进行四肢运动 [2]
Limb ataxia(肢体共济失调)	A kind of "ataxia" (HP:0001251) that affects movements of the extremities [2]
Limb ataxia(肢体共济失调)	影响肢体运动的一种共济失调（HP:0001251）[2]
Limb dysmetria(肢体辨距不良)	A type of "dysmetria" (HP:0001310) involving the limbs [2]
Limb dysmetria(肢体辨距不良)	累及肢体的一种辨距不良（HP:0001310）[2]
Limb dystonia(肢体肌张力障碍)	A type of dystonia (abnormally increased muscular tone causing fixed abnormal postures) that affects muscles of the limbs [2]
Limb dystonia(肢体肌张力障碍)	影响肢体肌肉的一种肌张力障碍（异常肌张力增加导致固定的异常姿势）[2]
Limb shaking TIA(肢体抖动性短暂性脑缺血发作)	A transient ischemic attack which is typically associated with severe large artery disease with exhausted hemodynamic reserve is "limb shaking TIA". It is characterized by 30–60 sec episodes of repetitive jerking movements of contralateral arm and/or leg and has been described with carotid occlusion but also with stenosis of intracranial vessels, e.g. middle cerebral artery or anterior cerebral artery. "Limb shaking TIA" is elicited in situations which dispose to low flow, e.g. orthostatic dysregulation, hyperventilation in Moyamoya disease, or by carotid compression [1]

续　表

英文术语（中文术语）	定义（英文和/或中文）
Line Bisection test(线段等分试验)	A simple task wherein the examinee is asked to draw a line that bisects lines of varying length. Diller, Ben-Yishay, and Gerstman (1974) presented a technique in which the examiner draws the line for the patient or instructs the patient to copy an already drawn horizontal line. The patient is then asked to divide the line in half by placing an "X" on the center point. Schenkenberg, Bradford and Ajax (1980) developed a multiple trial line bisection test that uses a set of 20 lines of varying sizes arranged so that six are centered to the left of the midline on a 8 ½ × 11 sheet of paper, six to the midline, and six in the center along with a top and bottom line to be used for instructions are centered on the page. The examiner then asks the patient to "Cut each line in half by placing a small pencil mark through each line as close to its center as possible." [1]
Lipid peroxidation(脂质过氧化)	Lipid peroxidation can be described generally as a process under which oxidants such as free radicals or nonradical species attack lipids containing carbon-carbon double bond(s), especially polyunsaturated fatty acids (PUFAs) that involve hydrogen abstraction from a carbon, with oxygen insertion resulting in lipid peroxyl radicals and hydroperoxides as described previously [1]
Lipohyalinosis(脂质玻璃样变)	Lipohyalinosis is a small-vessel disease in the brain. Originally defined by Fisher as "segmental arteriolar wall disorganisation", it is characterised by vessel wall thickening and a resultant reduction in luminal diameter. Fisher considered this small-vessel disease to be the result of hypertension, induced in the acute stage by fibrinoid necrosis that would lead to occlusion and hence lacunar stroke [1]
Lipoprotein associated phospholipase A2(脂蛋白相关磷酯酶A2)	A lipoprotein-associated PHOSPHOLIPASE A2 which modulates the action of PLATELET ACTIVATING FACTOR by hydrolyzing the SN-2 ester bond to yield the biologically inactive lyso-platelet-activating factor. It has specificity for phospholipid substrates with short-chain residues at the SN-2 position, but inactive against long-chain phospholipids. Deficiency in this enzyme is associated with many diseases including ASTHMA, and HYPERCHOLESTEROLEMIA [1]

英文术语（中文术语）	定义（英文和/或中文）
Locked in syndrome(闭锁综合征)	Locked in syndrome (LIS) is a condition that can occur as a result of a stroke involving the brainstem; the stroke damages the ventral brainstem, corresponding to the pyramidal bundles[1]
Logorrhea(多语症)	Logorrhea means excessive verbal production; it is manifested as an unusual verbosity that may suggest the presence of neurological or psychiatric pathologies[1]
Loss of corneal reflex(角膜反射减少)	An abnormally reduced response to stimulation of the cornea (by touch, foreign body, blowing air). The corneal reflex (also known as the blink reflex, normally results in an involuntary blinking of the eyelids[1]
Loss of pain(痛觉消失)	Reduced ability to perceive painful stimuli[2]
Loss of pain(痛觉消失)	感知疼痛刺激的能力下降[2]
Loss of temperature(温度觉障碍)	Temperature sensation can be tested by touching the skin several seconds with a water flask filled to the desired temperature. Persons with normal temperature sensation should at least be able to identify as warm a flask that is 35-36 degrees C and identify as cool a flask at 28-32 degrees C. A reduced ability to discriminate between different temperatures[1]
Low glycaemic index diet intake(低血糖指数饮食摄入)	Food with a high glycaemic index has been shown to increase the risk of mortality from stroke (ischaemic and haemorrhagic) in Japanese women and a higher dietary glycaemic load (GL) was associated with a greater risk of haemorrhagic stroke in Swedish middle-aged and older men, as well as an increased risk of total stroke, but not haemorrhagic stroke, in over-weight women[1]
Low molecular weight heparins(低分子肝素)	Low molecular weight heparins (LMWH) have been shown to have advantages over standard unfractionated heparins in the prevention of pulmonary embolism and, in this context, appear to have a better safety profile. There was, therefore, considerable hope that they would prove more efficacious in the treatment of acute stroke[1]
Low-to-normal blood pressure(血压低至正常)	Mild decrease of blood pressure[2]
Low-to-normal blood pressure(血压低至正常)	是指体循环动脉压力稍低于正常的状态[2]

续　表

英文术语（中文术语）	定义（英文和/或中文）
Lower extremity weakness(下肢无力)	Weakness of the muscles of the legs. Inability to perform rapid, alternating movements[1]
Lubeluzole(芦贝鲁唑)	The exact mechanism of action of lubeluzole, a drug effective in animal models, is unclear. The drug may block sodium channels in cells. In addition, it may reduce the release of nitric oxide, a neurotransmitter generated by activation of the NMDA receptor[1]
Magnesium(镁)	Magnesium is another agent with actions on the NMDA receptor and a low incidence of adverse effects. It may reduce ischemic injury by increasing regional blood flow, antagonizing voltage-sensitive calcium channels, and blocking the NMDA receptor[1]
Magnetic resonance angiography(磁共振血管成像)	Magnetic resonance angiography (MRA) is a set of vascular imaging techniques capable of depicting the extracranial and intracranial circulation[1]
Magnetic resonance angiography(磁共振血管成像)	Non-invasive method of vascular imaging and determination of internal anatomy without injection of contrast media or radiation exposure. The technique is used especially in CEREBRAL ANGIOGRAPHY as well as for studies of other vascular structures. A diagnostic technique for measuring the rate at which blood is delivered to tissue. In perfusion MRI, an exogenous contrast agent is usually injected to provide superior tissue contrast and easy delineation of perfusion abnormalities. Endogenous markers can also be used[1]
Magnetic resonance imaging(磁共振成像)	Non-invasive method of demonstrating internal anatomy based on the principle that atomic nuclei in a strong magnetic field absorb pulses of radiofrequency energy and emit them as radiowaves which can be reconstructed into computerized images. The concept includes proton spin tomographic techniques[1]
Malondialdehyde［丙二醛（MDA）］	The dialdehyde of malonic acid[1]
Mannitol(甘露醇)	Mannitol decreases blood viscosity, which results in reflex vasoconstriction and decreased cerebrovascular volume. The major problems associated with mannitol administration are hypovolemia and the induction of a hyperosmotic state[1]

英文术语（中文术语）	定义（英文和/或中文）
Marie Foix syndrome(脑桥外侧综合征)	Lateral pontine syndrome, also known as Marie-Foix syndrome, refers to one of the brainstem stroke syndromes which occurs due to occlusion of perforating branches of the basilar and anterior inferior cerebellar (AICA) arteries. This results in infarction of the lateral aspect of the pons which produces characteristic clinical picture from involvement of the following pontine structures: -corticospinal tract leads to contralateral hemiplegia/hemiparesis. -spinothalamic tract causes contralateral loss of pain and temperature sensation. -cerebellar tracts causes ipsilteral limb ataxia. -CN VII nucleus leads to ipsilateral facial paralysis. -CN VIII vestibular and cochlear nuclei leads to ipsilateral hearing loss, vertigo and nystagmus[1]
Mast cell expressed membrane protein 1(肥大细胞表达膜蛋白1)	Mast cell expressed membrane protein 1 (MCEMP1), also known as C19ORF59, is a transmembrane protein expressed by mast cells,24 macrophages and other tissues[1]
Mathew stroke scale(马修卒中量表)	The Mathew Stroke Scale was originally designed to test neurologic deficit as part of an acute stroke study testing the therapeutic efficacy of glycerol[1]
Matrix metalloproteinase 1(基质金属蛋白酶1)	A member of the metalloproteinase family of enzymes that is principally responsible for cleaving FIBRILLAR COLLAGEN. It can degrade interstitial collagens, types I, II and III[1]
Matrix metalloproteinase 13〔基质金属蛋白酶13(MMP-13)〕	A secreted matrix metalloproteinase that plays a physiological role in the degradation of extracellular matrix found in skeletal tissues. It is synthesized as an inactive precursor that is activated by the proteolytic cleavage of its N-terminal propeptide[1]
Matrix metalloproteinase 2(基质金属蛋白酶2)	A secreted endopeptidase homologous with INTERSTITIAL COLLAGENASE, but which possesses an additional fibronectin-like domain[1]
Matrix metalloproteinase 3(基质金属蛋白酶3)	An extracellular endopeptidase of vertebrate tissues similar to MATRIX METALLOPROTEINASE 1. It digests PROTEOGLYCAN; FIBRONECTIN; COLLAGEN types III, IV, V, and IX, and activates procollagenase. (Enzyme Nomenclature, 1992)[1]

续 表

英文术语（中文术语）	定义（英文和/或中文）
Matrix metalloproteinase 9(基质金属蛋白酶9)	An endopeptidase that is structurally similar to MATRIX METALLOPROTEINASE 2. It degrades GELATIN types I and V; COLLAGEN TYPE IV; and COLLAGEN TYPE V [1]
Matrix metalloproteinases(基质金属蛋白酶)	MMPs are a family of 14 enzymes, a subset of which have been found to be active in brain tissue. The various MMPs function as stromelysines, gelatinases, colagenases, a membrane-type proteinase and a matrilysin [1]
Measures of comorbidity(共病措施)	In epidemiology, a rating scale for comorbidity [1]
Mechanical Clot Disruption(机械性血栓破裂)	Mechanical approaches to arterial recanalization using balloons, snares, or the embolectomy devices have been reported with promising results [1]
Mechanical Clot Extraction(机械性血栓提取)	Devices have been used to extract thrombi from occluded intracranial arteries [1]
Mechanisms of atherosclerotic cerebrovascular disease(动脉粥样硬化性脑血管病的发病机制)	Three basic mechanisms can result in cessation or diminution of flow to regions of brain: embolism from a proximal source with occlusion of the downstream artery; local occlusion, usually due to in situ thrombosis, of a proximal or distal artery; or global hypoperfusion [1]
Medial medullary infarction symptom(延髓内侧综合征)	The medial medullary stroke is a rare stroke syndrome and classically includes contralateral hemiparesis sparing the face (corticospinal tract), contralateral lemniscal sensory loss (medial lemniscus) and ipsilateral tongue paresis (nucleus of hypoglossal nerve and tract) [1]
Mediterranean diet(地中海饮食)	The Mediterranean diet is a collection of eating habits traditionally followed by people in the diff erent countries bordering the Mediterranean Sea. This diet is characterised by a high consumption of fruit, vegetables, legumes, and complex carbohydrates (whole grains); a moderate consumption of fi sh; consumption of olive oil as the main source of fats (monounsaturated); a low-to-moderate amount of red wine during meals; and low consumption of red meat, refi ned grains, and sweets [1]

英文术语（中文术语）	定义（英文和/或中文）
Mediterranean diet(地中海饮食)	There is no single definition of a Mediterranean diet, but such diets are typically high in fruits, vegetables, whole grains, beans, nuts, and seeds; include olive oil as an important source of monounsaturated fat; and allow low to moderate wine consumption. There are typically low to moderate amounts of fish, poultry, and dairy products, with little red meat. The Mediterranean diet is associated with several health benefits; however, it remains uncertain which components of the Mediterranean diet offer the protective benefit or if the benefits result from an aggregation of effects [1]
melodic intonation therapy(旋律语调疗法)	通过非优势侧半球的旋律训练，使辅助言语功能被活化，以改善言语功能的训练方法。训练时，用一些富有旋律的句子做吟诵训练，使患者学会使用夸张的韵律、重音、旋律来表达正常的语言 [3]
Metabolic disease(代谢性疾病)	Generic term for diseases caused by an abnormal metabolic process. It can be congenital due to inherited enzyme abnormality (METABOLISM, INBORN ERRORS) or acquired due to disease of an endocrine organ or failure of a metabolically important organ such as the liver. (Stedman, 26th ed) [1]
Metabolic syndrome(代谢综合征)	The metabolic syndrome is associated with a higher risk of CVD, including stroke. According to criteria of the National Cholesterol Education Program Adult Treatment Panel III (ATP III), diagnosis of metabolic syndrome is made when of the following risk factors are present: abdominal obesity, elevated triglyceride levels, low levels of high-density lipoprotein cholesterol (HDL-C), elevated blood pressure, and impaired glucose metabolism [1]
Metamorphopsia(视物变形)	General term for a range of visual perceptual disorders in which the apparent shape, size, outline, color, number, movement, or other physical characteristics of visual objects are distorted [1]
Microcirculatory dysfunction(微循环障碍)	The hypothesis that the cerebral microcirculation has to be involved in posthemorrhagic cerebral ischemia was based on experimental studies showing that acutely following SAH intracranial pressure increased so dramatically that CBF (and in parallel CPP) decrease to almost zero thereby causing global cerebral ischemia [1]

英文术语（中文术语）	定义（英文和/或中文）
Midbrain infarction symptom(中脑梗死综合征)	The arterial blood supply to the midbrain is complex. Infarcts limited to the midbrain are uncommon and usually are accompanied by involvement of other structures such as the cerebellum, thalamus,andpons[1]
Middle cereberal artery infarction syndrome (大脑中动脉梗死综合征)	The middle cerebral artery (MCA) is also designated the Sylvian artery, from Jacques Dubois, known as Jacobus Sylvius (1489–1555), a linguist and anatomist in Paris. The artery is subdivided into the M1 segment, from which start the deep perforating lenticulostriate arteries, the M2 segment, corresponding to the segment after the bifurcation into superior and inferior divisions, and the M3 segment, including the insular part. The M4 segments, the leptomeningeal arteries, arise from the M3 segments and are named orbitofrontal, prefrontal, precentral, central sulcus, anterior parietal, posterior parietal, angular and temporal arteries, with important variations in their territories. The MCA territory is the one most frequently affected by acute strokes. MCA territory infarcts can be subtle or a devastating clinical syndrome, depending on the site of the occlusion, the extent of ischemia, the etiology, and the collateral arterial network. As collateral networks are highly variable, an occlusion of the same artery at the same place may lead to quite variable severity of the stroke and of prognosis. Large infarcts are defined as involvement of two of the three MCA territories (deep, superior and inferior divisions) and "malignant MCA stroke" as complete or near complete MCA territory infarction with ensuing mass effect from brain edema[1]
Migraine(偏头痛)	Migraine is a chronic neurological disorder characterized by episodic attacks of headache and associated symptoms[2]
Migraine(偏头痛)	偏头痛是一种慢性神经系统疾病，特点是发作性头痛及相关症状[2]

续　表

英文术语（中文术语）	定义（英文和/或中文）
Migraine with aura(先兆偏头痛)	A type of "migraine" (HP:0002076) in which there is an aura characterized by focal neurological phenomena that usually proceed, but may accompany or occur in the absence of, the headache. The symptoms of an aura may include fully reversible visual, sensory, and speech symptoms but not motor weakness. Visual symptoms may include flickering lights, spots and lines and/or loss of vision and/or unilateral sensory symptoms such as paresthesias or numbness. At least one of the symptoms of an aura develops gradually over 5 or more minutes and/or different symptoms occur in succession[2]
Migraine with aura(先兆偏头痛)	偏头痛（HP:0002076）的一种类型，先兆的特点为局灶性神经现象，通常进行性的，可伴有或不伴有头痛。先兆的症状可以包括完全可逆的视觉，感觉，和言语症状，但没有运动无力。视觉症状可能包括闪光、点、线和/或视觉缺失，和/或单侧感觉症状诸如感觉异常或麻木。至少一个的先兆症状逐渐发展超过5分钟或更长时间，和/或不同的症状连续发生[2]
Migraine without aura(无先兆偏头痛)	Repeated headache attacks lasting 4-72 h fulfilling at least two of the following criteria: 1) unilateral location, 2) pulsating quality, 3) moderate or severe pain intensity, and 4) aggravation by or causing avoidance of routine physical activity such as climbing stairs. Headache attacks are commonly accompanied by nausea, vomiting, photophobia, or phonophobia[2]
Migraine without aura(无先兆偏头痛)	反复的头痛发作持续4-72小时，符合至少下列两个的标准:1）单侧，2）搏动性，3）中度或重度疼痛，4）日常体力活动可加重，避免日常活动如爬楼梯。头痛发作通常伴有恶心，呕吐，畏光，或畏声[2]
Migrainous infarction(偏头痛性脑梗死)	Migraine is a neurological disease associated with an increased stroke risk[1]
Migrainous infarction(偏头痛性脑梗死)	Migraine is a neurological disease associated with an increased stroke risk[1]
Millard Gubler syndrome(脑桥腹外侧综合征)	Millard Gubler syndrome, also known as ventral pontine syndrome, is one of the crossed paralysis syndromes, which are characterised by cranial nerves VI and VII palsies with contralateral body motor or sensory disturbances[1]

续　表

英文术语（中文术语）	定义（英文和/或中文）
Minocycline(米诺环素)	minocycline appears to decrease levels of matrix metalloproteinase-9, which has been associated with recombinant tissue plasminogen activator (rtPA)–associated cerebral hemorrhage[1]
Miosis(瞳孔缩小)	Contraction of the pupil or condition in which the pupil is very small (2 mm or less in diameter). It can be brought about by a spasm of the sphincter muscle or by the effect of a miotic drug (e.g. eserine, neostigmine, pilocarpine), or in certain spinal diseases or any stimulation of the parasympathetic supply to the eye. Miosis occurs naturally when doing close work or when stimulated by light[1]
Mitochondrial cytopathy(线粒体细胞病)	Mitochondrial cytopathies represent a heterogeneous group of multisystem disorders which preferentially affect the muscle and nervous systems. They are caused either by mutations in the maternally inherited mitochondrial genome, or by nuclear DNA-mutations[1]
Modified Rankin Scale(改良 Rankin 量表)	The modified Rankin Scale (mRS) consists of six levels of classification that describe the degree of disability in stroke survivors[1]
monocarboxylic acid transporter(单羧酸转运体)	A family of proteins involved in the transport of monocarboxylic acids such as LACTIC ACID and PYRUVIC ACID across cellular membranes[1]
Monoclonal antibodies(单克隆抗体类)	Monoclonal antibodies can block an intercellular adhesion molecule (ICAM) on the endothelium to prevent adhesion of white blood cells to the vessel wall. Because anti-ICAM antibodies appear to block an early step in reperfusion-related injury, they present a hopeful mechanism for preserving neuronal function[1]
Monocular horizontal nystagmus(单眼水平性眼球震颤)	Monocular horizontal nystagmus[2]
Monocular horizontal nystagmus(单眼水平性眼球震颤)	单眼水平性的眼球震颤[2]

英文术语（中文术语）	定义（英文和/或中文）
Monocyte chemoattractant protein 1(单核细胞趋化因子-1)	A chemokine that is a chemoattractant for MONOCYTES and may also cause cellular activation of specific functions related to host defense. It is produced by LEUKOCYTES of both monocyte and lymphocyte lineage and by FIBROBLASTS during tissue injury. It has specificity for CCR2 RECEPTORS[1]
Motor Assessment Scale(运动评估量表)	The Motor Assessment Scale (MAS) is a performance based scale that assesses everyday motor function in patients with stroke (Carr et al., 1985) and other neurological impairments. It is a task-oriented approach to evaluation that assesses performance of functional tasks rather than isolated patterns of movement (Malouin et al., 1994). It evaluates a patient's ability to move with low muscle tone or in a synergistic or stereotypical upper motor neuron pattern and to move actively out of that pattern into normal movement[1]
motor dysfunction(运动障碍)	Motor deficits are among the most common manifestations in patients with ACA-territory infarctions. In classic descriptions, cortical branch occlusion usually results in motor deficits of the foot and leg and, to a lesser degree, paresis of the arm, with the face and tongue largely spared[1]
Motor Evaluation Scale for Upper Extremity in Stroke Patients(脑卒中患者上肢运动评价量表)	The MESUPES arm and hand tests are the first scales that take quality of movement into account when documenting upper limb function in stroke patients. Both scales cover a range of items focusing on tone adaptation, selective movement and complicated functional tasks[1]
Motor hemineglect(运动性忽略症)	Motor hemineglect is characterized by an underutilization of one side of the body. It is a higher-order motor disorder that resembles hemiplegia although being substantially different from it due to a preserved motor output system[1]
Motor-Free Visual Perception Test(无运动视觉感知测试)	Designed to assess an individual's "visual perceptual ability without any motor involvement needed to make a response."[1]

续　表

英文术语（中文术语）	定义（英文和/或中文）
Moyamoya disease(烟雾病)	MOYAMOYA, a Japanese word meaning "something hazy like a puff of cigarette smoke drifting in the air," is the descriptive term we apply to a peculiar angiographic picture consisting of abnormal net-like vessels at the base of the brain. In addition to this abnormality, angiography usually reveals stenosis or occlusion of the internal carotid artery at the level of its terminal bifurcation together with abnormalities of the anterior and middle cerebral arteries. These changes are usually bilateral[1]
Moyamoya disease(烟雾病)	Moyamoya syndrome is a disease in which certain arteries in the brain are constricted. Blood flow is blocked by the constriction, and also by blood clots[1]
Multimodal reperfusion therapy(多模式再灌注治疗)	The MMRT approach is particularly promising for patients with anterior circulation infarcts. MMRT, including mechanical thrombolysis, IA lytic drugs, clot retrievers and angioplasty with stenting, increases the chances of reperfusion in these patients[1]
Multiple sclerosis(多发性硬化)	Multiple sclerosis (MS) is a chronic inflammatory demyelinating disease of the central nervous system (CNS) affecting the brain and spinal cord[1]
Myelin basic protein(髓鞘碱性蛋白)	Myelin basic protein (MBP) is a hydrophilic protein important for the correct structure of myelin sheaths[1]
Myoclonic spasms(肌阵挛性抽搐)	Marked by a sudden contraction of a muscle or muscle mass, resulting in sudden, rapid twitching of the face, trunk, or limbs[2]
Myoclonic spasms(肌阵挛性抽搐)	表现为某个肌肉或肌群的突然收缩，引起面、躯干或肢体突然快速的抽动[2]
Myoclonus(肌阵挛)	Myoclonus is exceptionally seen in patients with strokes, outside of clonic seizures. Generalized myoclonus has never been reported. The anoxic action myoclonus of Lance & Adams (1963) has been reported in association with multiple lacunar lesions in the basal ganglia. Intention and action myoclonus was found in a patient with a thalamic angioma. Focal reflex myoclonus has been reported by Sutton & Meyer (1974) in a patient with a superficial sylvian stroke involving the frontoparietal lobes and later by others[1]

续　表

英文术语（中文术语）	定义（英文和/或中文）
Myoclonus(肌阵挛)	Very brief, involuntary random muscular contractions occurring at rest, in response to sensory stimuli, or accompanying voluntary movements[2]
Myoclonus(肌阵挛)	很简短，随意不自主的肌肉收缩发生在休息，以应对感官刺激，或陪同随意运动[2]
N acetylaspartate(N乙酰天冬氨酸)	N-acetylaspartate (NAA) is a free amino acid representing approximately 1% of the dry weight of the brain[1]
N formyl peptide receptor(N甲酰肽受体)	A rhodopsin-like G-protein coupled receptor that is a translation product of the FPR1, FPR2, or FPR3 gene and whose active form binds N-formyl methionyl peptides[1]
N glycan(N聚糖)	N-glycans are oligosaccharide structures covalently linked (sugar–amino acid linkage) to an asparagine residue of a protein in a consensus sequence (GlcNAc-b-Asn). These sugar structures are highly heterogeneous and their biosynthesis is closely linked to the cellular metabolism, thereby they reflect the metabolic status of cells[1]
N terminal proBNP(N末端脑钠肽前体)	A bioassay to determine an individual's level of N-terminal pro-brain natriuretic peptide (NT-proBNP)[1]
Nalmefene(纳美芬)	Nalmefene (Cervene) is a narcotic receptor antagonist that reduces levels of excitatory neurotransmitters contributing to cellular injury in early ischemia[1]
Nasal, dysarthic speech(鼻，构音障碍)	Speech impairment due to neuropathy, speech-related muscle paralysis, decreased contractility, or lack of motor coordination[2]
Nasal, dysarthic speech(鼻，构音障碍)	由于神经病变，与言语有关的肌肉麻痹、收缩力减弱或运动不协调所致的言语障碍[2]

续 表

英文术语（中文术语）	定义（英文和/或中文）
National Institutes of Health Stroke Scale(美国国立卫生研究院卒中量表)	The National Institutes of Health Stroke Scale (NIHSS) is a score calculated from 11 components and is used to quantify the severity of strokes. The 11 components are: level of consciousness (1a: 0-3, 1b: 0-2 and 1c: 0-2) best gaze (0-2) visual fields (0-3) facial palsy (0-3) arm motor (0-4) leg motor (0-4) limb ataxia (0-2) sensory (0-2) best language (0-3) dysarthria (0-2) extinction and inattention (0-2) These 11 components are then summed and the score correlates with stroke severity. 0 = no stroke symptoms 1-4 = minor stroke 5-15 = moderate stroke 16-20 = moderate to severe stroke 21-42 = severe stroke[1]
Nausea(恶心)	A sensation of unease in the stomach together with an urge to vomit[1]
Neurochemical changes(神经化学改变)	Postmortem (by immunohistochemical staining techniques) and in vivo (by microdialysis) evaluation of neurochemical changes following stroke in animal models showed that while aspartate, glutamate, inosine, hypoxanthine, adenosine and γ-aminobutyrate increases in the acute ischemic period, glycine seems to increase with prolonged ischemia and some neuroactive substances increase in peri-infarct region (such as tyrosine hydroxylase, neuropeptide Y), and some (neuropeptide Y, leuleuenkephalin, neurotensin, and dynorphin) in nuclei of amygdala which are not infarcted[1]
Neurofilament light protein(神经丝轻蛋白)	Nurofilament is a triplet protein that forms part of the structural scaffold of neurons. Neurofilament light protein (NFL) is the subunit that forms the core of the filament. Increased levels of NFL have been observed in a variety of neurodegenerative diseases. Increased CSF concentration of NFL has also been shown in a small series of patients following ischemic stroke[1]
Neurogenic bladder(神经源性膀胱)	Dysfunction of the URINARY BLADDER due to disease of the central or peripheral nervous system pathways involved in the control of URINATION. This is often associated with SPINAL CORD DISEASES, but may also be caused by BRAIN DISEASES or PERIPHERAL NERVE DISEASES[1]

英文术语（中文术语）	定义（英文和/或中文）
Neuroimaging(神经影像学)	Non-invasive methods of visualizing the CENTRAL NERVOUS SYSTEM, especially the brain, by various imaging modalities[1]
Neuroimaging biomarkers of stroke(脑卒中的神经影像学生物标志物)	Neuroimaging is widely used to aid in the diagnosis of stroke, to assist in determining a likely etiology for the event, to estimate severity, and to predict functional outcome and risk of recurrence[1]
Neurone specific enolase(神经元特异性烯醇化酶)	Neuron-specific enolase is one of three recognized forms of enolase, an enzyme in the glycolysis pathway[1]
Neuroprotective therapy(神经保护治疗)	Neuroprotective agents are used in an attempt to save ischemic neurons in the brain from irreversible injury[1]
Neuroserpin(神经源性丝氨酸蛋白酶抑制剂)	Neuroserpin is a serine protease inhibitor (serpin) that selectively inhibits tissue plasminogen activator (tPA) within the central nervous system (CNS). Neuroserpin is secreted by neurons in the brain, and provides regulation of tPA activity during both normal and pathological processes including CNS development, neuronal survival, and cerebral ischemia[1]
Nimodipine(尼莫地平)	stroke among persons with recent aneurysmal subarachnoid hemorrhage[1]
Nitric oxide(一氧化氮)	Nitric oxide (NO) has one unpaired electron and can be regarded ass a free radical. NO generation and its reactive products with oxygen free radicals may be highly cytotoxxic[1]
NMDA autoantibodies(N-甲基D-天冬氨酸自身抗体)	The NMDA glutamine receptor is implicated in mediating the excitotoxic response in cerebral ischemia. Autoantibodies (aAbs) to the NR2 subtype of the NMDA receptor have been demonstrated to be associated with neurotoxicity[1]
Noncontrast MRA(非对比MRA)	MRA is broadly divided into noncontrast and contrast-enhanced techniques.Noncontrast MRA can be acquired with phase contrast (PC) or TOF techniques, and both can be acquired as 2D slabs or 3D volumes[1]
Nonspecifc markers of coagulation(凝血相关非特异性标志物)	Some coagulation markers have been used extensively for diagnostic purposes for other conditions. The limitation to the use of coagulation markers is that they are nonspecifc in nature[1]

续　表

英文术语（中文术语）	定义（英文和/或中文）
Nuclear factor kappa B(核转录因子-kB)	Nuclear factor-κB is a ubiquitous transcription factor that is a critical regulator of numerous responses including inflammation (Barnes, 1996) and pro-inflammatory genes such as TNF-α, IL-1β, nitric oxide synthase, HO-1 and intracellular adhesion molecule-1[1]
Nucleoside diphosphate kinase A(核苷二磷酸激酶a亚基)	NDKA is a kinase that catalyzes the transfer of the terminal phosphate from ATP to nucleotides[1]
Nucleoside diphosphate kinase A(核苷二磷酸激酶a亚基)	Nucleoside diphosphate kinase A (152 aa, ~17 kDa) is encoded by the human NME1 gene. This protein plays a role in nucleoside triphosphate synthesis, lipid and protein phosphorylation, apoptosis and the regulation of cell proliferation[1]
Nucleosomes(核小体)	Nucleosomes are cell death products that are elevated in serum of patients with diseases that are associated with massive cell destruction. The kinetics of circulating nucleosomes after cerebral stroke and their correlation with the clinical status have been investigated[1]
Nystagmus(眼球震颤)	Rhythmic, involuntary oscillations of one or both eyes related to abnormality in fixation, conjugate gaze, or vestibular mechanisms[2]
Nystagmus(眼球震颤)	一种规律性，非自主的单眼或双眼震颤，震颤的双眼不能固视、共轭凝视，或前庭病变[2]
Nystagmus-induced head nodding(眼球震颤诱发的点头运动)	Head movements associated with nystagmus, that may represent an attempt to compensate for the involuntary eye movements and to improve vision[2]
Nystagmus-induced head nodding(眼球震颤诱发的点头运动)	头的活动与眼球震颤相联系，这可能是企图以头颅的运动代偿眼球不自主运动，提高视力[2]
Obesity(肥胖)	A status with BODY WEIGHT that is grossly above the acceptable or desirable weight, usually due to accumulation of excess FATS in the body. The standards may vary with age, sex, genetic or cultural background. In the BODY MASS INDEX, a BMI greater than 30.0 kg/m2 is considered obese, and a BMI greater than 40.0 kg/m2 is considered morbidly obese (MORBID OBESITY)[1]

续 表

英文术语（中文术语）	定义（英文和/或中文）
Obstructive sleep apnea(阻塞性睡眠呼吸暂停综合症)	Apneas or hypopneas resulting from complete or partial collapse of the upper airway collapse during sleep. This is the mostcommon type of SDB in patients with acute cerebrovascular disorders. Although patients at risk for cerebrovascular disease frequently have OSA before they experience a stroke, in some patients OSA appears to have been aggravated (e.g. by sleep disruption, Cheyne–Stokes breathing) or even caused "de novo" (e.g. medullary infarction, severe pharyngeal palsy) by acute brain ischemia[1]
Occipital neuralgia(枕神经痛)	A distinct type of headache characterized by piercing, throbbing, or electric-shock-like chronic pain in the upper neck, back of the head, and behind the ears, usually on one side[2]
Occipital neuralgia(枕神经痛)	一种明显的以尖锐性、抽动性或电击样疼痛为特征的慢性头痛，通常存在于一侧的上颈部、后头部或耳后[2]
Occupational Therapy Adult Perceptual Screening Test(职业治疗成人知觉筛查试验)	The OT-APST was designed to comprehensively screen for the most commonly occurring changes in visual perception following stroke and other acquired brain injuries affecting adults. It is recommended for use in combination with skilled occupational analysis of daily life tasks and can assist the occupational therapist to determine the separate contributions of visual perceptual impairments and apraxia to functional task performance[1]
Ocular dyssynergia(眼协同失调)	A type of "dyssynergia" (HP:0010867) affecting eye movements and characterized by the inability to smoothly follow a visual target across the visual field[2]
Ocular dyssynergia(眼协同失调)	一种影响眼球运动的以无法流畅的在视野中追踪物体为特征的眼协同失调[2]
Ocular tilt reaction(眼倾斜反应)	An ocular tilt reaction is characterized by the triad of skew deviation (downward displacement of the axis of the globe ipsilateral to the lesion), conjugate ocular torsion towards the side of the lesion and head tilt to the side of the lesion[1]

续　表

英文术语（中文术语）	定义（英文和/或中文）
Oculogyric crisis(动眼危象)	An acute dystonic reaction with blepharospasm, periorbital twitches, and protracted fixed staring episodes. There may be a maximal upward deviation of the eyes in the sustained fashion. Oculogyric crisis can be triggered by a number of factors including neuroleptic medications[2]
Oculogyric crisis(动眼危象)	眼睑痉挛，眶周抽搐，和长期固定注视的一种急性肌张力障碍，可能伴有持续的眼球最大向上运动的偏差。动眼神经危象可被很多因素包括镇静药物所诱发[2]
Oculomotor apraxia(眼球运动不能)	faulty visual scanning with an inability to project gaze voluntarily into the peripheral field and scan it despite full eye movements[1]
Oculomotor apraxia(眼球运动不能)	Inability to follow objects visually with compensatory head movements, decreased smooth pursuit, and cancellation of the vestibulo-ocular reflex[2]
Oculomotor apraxia(眼球运动不能)	即使有代偿性头运动，也无法直观地跟随物体，平滑移动减弱，前庭眼反射消失[2]
Ondine syndrome(Ondine综合征)	Ondine's curse is a rare and severe condition and is characterized by loss of automatic respiration during sleep and preserved voluntary breathing[1]
Onset of symptom(开始出现症状)	The single most important piece of historical information is the time of symptom onset. The current definition of the time of stroke onset is when patients were at their previous baseline or symptom-free state[1]
Ontario Society of Occupational Therapists Perceptual Evaluation(安大略职业治疗师学会感性评估)	The OSOT Perceptual Evaluation consists of 28 tests organized under the following six functional areas: Sensory Function, Scanning and Spatial Neglect, Apraxia, Body Awareness, Spatial Relations, and Visual Agnosia[1]
Optic ataxia(视觉性共济失调)	Optic ataxia is a deficit of visually guided hand movements toward a normally perceived object in the peripheral visual field(s)[1]

英文术语（中文术语）	定义（英文和/或中文）
Optokinetic nystagmus(视旋转性眼球震颤)	The optokinetic reflex is a combination of a saccade and smooth pursuit eye movements. It is seen when an individual follows a moving object with their eyes, which then moves out of the field of vision at which point their eye moves back to the position it was in when it first saw the object. The reflex develops at about 6 months of age [1]
Orgogozo stroke scale(奥戈佐卒中量表)	The Orgogozo Scale includes assessments of consciousness, language and motor function [1]
Oromandibular dystonia(口下颌肌张力障碍)	A kind of focal dystonia characterized by forceful contractions of the face, jaw, and/or tongue causing difficulty in opening and closing the mouth and often affecting chewing and speech [2]
Oromandibular dystonia(口下颌肌张力障碍)	一种局限性肌张力障碍，表现为脸，下颌，和/或舌的有力的收缩导致难以打开和关闭嘴部和经常影响咀嚼和讲话 [2]
orosomucoid 1(血清类黏蛋白1)	ORM1, also known as α-1 acid glycoprotein, is an acute phase protein that suppresses lymphocyte response to lipopolysaccharides (thereby preventing ongoing tissue damage by neutrophil proteases), decreases platelet aggregation (and further platelet recruitment), and enhances cytokine secretion [1]
Orpington Prognostic Scale(奥平顿预后量表)	The Orpington Prognostic Scale and the NIH Stroke Scale were used to measure stroke severity at baseline. The Orpington Prognostic Scale includes measures of motor deficit in arm, proprioception, balance, and cognition [1]
Orthostatic hypotension(体位性低血压)	A form of hypotension characterized by a sudden fall in blood pressure that occurs when a person assumes a standing position [2]
Orthostatic hypotension(体位性低血压)	当一个人变换为站立位时血压突然下降的一种低血压 [2]
Orthostatic syncope(直立性晕厥)	Syncope following a quick change in position from lying down to standing [2]
Orthostatic syncope(直立性晕厥)	从躺着到站起，突然的体位变化引起的晕厥 [2]

205

续　表

英文术语（中文术语）	定义（英文和/或中文）
Oxfordshire Community Stroke Project(Oxford 卒中分类)	The Bamford classification divides people with stroke into four different categories, according to the symptoms and signs with which they present. This classification is useful for understanding the likely underlying pathology, which in turn gives information on treatments likely to be useful and the prognosis. It is a relatively simple, robust, bedside classification using clinical information. This clinical tool categorizes stroke syndromes into 4 subtypes: total anterior circulation infarcts (TACI), partial anterior circulation infarcts (PACI), lacunar infarcts (LACI), and posterior circulation infarcts (POCI)[1]
Pain insensitivity(痛觉缺失)	Inability to perceive painful stimuli[2]
Pain insensitivity(痛觉缺失)	不能感知疼痛刺激[2]
Palatal myoclonus(软腭阵挛)	Palatal myoclonus is characterized by myoclonic (rhythmic involuntary jerky) movements of the soft palate[2]
Palatal myoclonus(软腭阵挛)	腭肌阵挛的特点是软腭的肌阵挛（节奏不自主跳动）动作[2]
Palatal weakness(腭部无力)	weakness of the muscles of the hard and soft palate[1]
Palinopsia(视像存留)	One of a variety of metamorphopsias in which a visual image either persists or recurs even after the original stimulus is no longer present[1]
Palipsychism(心理学)	a state of parallel expression of mental activities[1]
paramedian artery infarction symptom(旁动脉梗死症状)	The paramedian arteries arise from the P1 segment of the PCA. The inferior and middle rami irrigate parts of the midbrain and the pons, while the superior ramus irrigates a variable extent of thalamus but mostly the dorsomedial nucleus, the intralaminar nuclei and internal medullary lamina. Infarctions also tend to involve the medial midbrain[1]

英文术语（中文术语）	定义（英文和/或中文）
Paraoxonase 1(对氧磷酶1)	An enzyme which catalyzes the hydrolysis of an aryl-dialkyl phosphate to form dialkyl phosphate and an aryl alcohol. It can hydrolyze a broad spectrum of organophosphate substrates and a number of aromatic carboxylic acid esters. It may also mediate an enzymatic protection of LOW DENSITY LIPOPROTEINS against oxidative modification and the consequent series of events leading to ATHEROMA formation. The enzyme was previously regarded to be identical with Arylesterase (EC 3.1.1.2) [1]
Paresthesia(感觉异常)	Abnormal sensations such as tingling, pricking, or numbness of the skin with no apparent physical cause [2]
Paresthesia(感觉异常)	异常感觉如刺痛，穿刺，或皮肤的麻木，没有明显的物理生理原因 [2]
PARK 7(帕金森病蛋白7)	A protein that is a translation product of the human PARK7 gene or a 1:1 ortholog thereof [1]
PARK 7(帕金森病蛋白7)	PARK7 is a redox-sensitive molecular chaperone activated in the context of oxidative stress [1]
Paroxysmal choreoathetosis(发作性舞蹈手足徐动症)	Episodes of choreoathetosis that can occur following triggers such as quick voluntary movements [2]
Paroxysmal choreoathetosis(发作性舞蹈手足徐动症)	舞蹈手足徐动可能被出现以下动作如快速随意运动所触发 [2]
Paroxysmal dystonia(阵发性肌张力障碍)	A form of dystonia characterized by episodes of dystonia (often hemidystonia or generalized) lasting from minutes to hours. There are no dystonic symptoms between episodes [2]
Paroxysmal dystonia(阵发性肌张力障碍)	肌张力障碍的一种形式特征是肌张力障碍（通常偏身或全身），从几分钟到几个小时持续发作。有发作之间没有肌张力障碍的症状 [2]
Paroxysmal vertigo(阵发性眩晕)	Paroxysmal episodes of vertigo [2]
Pathophysiology of Atherosclerotic cerebro-vascular disease(动脉粥样硬化性脑血管病的病理生理学)	The pathophysiology of any disease is how the normal physiology is altered by a disease, or pathologic, process [1]
Pendular nystagmus(钟摆样眼球震颤)	Rhythmic, involuntary sinusoidal oscillations of one or both eyes. The waveform of pendular nystagmus may occur in any direction [2]

续　表

英文术语（中文术语）	定义（英文和/或中文）
Pendular nystagmus(钟摆样眼球震颤)	一个或两个眼睛有节奏的、不自主的正弦振荡。摆动性眼球震颤的波形可能发生在任何方向[2]
Perfusion weighted magnetic resonance imaging(灌注加权磁共振成像)	A diagnostic procedure to assess the circulatory perfusion of an anatomical location using a magnetic resonance imaging machine[1]
Pericentral scotoma(旁中心暗点)	A scotoma (area of diminished vision within the visual field) that surrounds the central fixation point[2]
Pericentral scotoma(旁中心暗点)	盲点（视野内视力减弱的区域）围绕中央固定点[2]
Peripheral visual field constriction with 10-20 degrees central field preserved(周边视野缩小且保留10-20度中心视野)	Peripheral visual field constriction with 10-20 degrees central field preserved[2]
Peripheral visual field constriction with 10-20 degrees central field preserved(周边视野缩小且保留10-20度中心视野)	周边视野缩小且保留10-20度中心视野[2]
Peripheral visual field constriction with 20-30 degrees central field preserved(周边视野缩小且保留20-30度中心视野)	Peripheral visual field constriction with 20-30 degrees central field preserved[2]
Peripheral visual field constriction with 20-30 degrees central field preserved(周边视野缩小且保留20-30度中心视野)	周边视野缩小且保留20-30度中心视野[2]
Peripheral visual field constriction with 30-40 degrees central field preserved(周边视野缩小且保留30-40度中心视野)	Peripheral visual field constriction with 30-40 degrees central field preserved[2]
Peripheral visual field constriction with 30-40 degrees central field preserved(周边视野缩小且保留30-40度中心视野)	周边视野缩小且保留30-40度中心视野[2]
Peripheral visual field constriction with 40-50 degrees central field preserved(周边视野缩小且保留40-50度中心视野)	Peripheral visual field constriction with 40-50 degrees central field preserved[2]
Peripheral visual field constriction with 40-50 degrees central field preserved(周边视野缩小且保留40-50度中心视野)	周边视野缩小且保留40-50度中心视野[2]

英文术语（中文术语）	定义（英文和/或中文）
Peripheral visual field constriction with >50 degrees central field preserved(周边视野缩小且保留 >50度中心视野)	A diminution of the peripheral visual field whereby at least 50 degrees of central field are preserved in all meridians [2]
Peripheral visual field constriction with >50 degrees central field preserved(周边视野缩小且保留 >50度中心视野)	周边视野缩小且保留至少50度的中心视野[2]
Peripheral visual field constriction with<10 degrees central field preserved(周边视野缩小且保留 <10度中心视野)	Peripheral visual field constriction with <10 degrees central field preserved [2]
Peripheral visual field constriction with<10 degrees central field preserved(周边视野缩小且保留 <10度中心视野)	周边视野缩小且保留 <10度中心视野[2]
Peripheral visual field loss(周边视野缺损)	Loss of peripheral vision with retention of central vision, resulting in a constricted circular tunnel-like field of vision [2]
Peripheral visual field loss(周边视野缺损)	周边视觉损失，中央视力保留，造成管状视野[2]
Pharynx and vocal cord weakness(咽喉和声带无力)	The vocal cord and pharyngeal weakness can be present at the onset of the distal-extremity weakness. At first, the voice has a hypophonic, breathy quality, but this may slowly progress to a wet, gurgling, hoarse voice with hypernasal resonance and difficulty with swallowing and aspiration. Activities such as gargling become impossible [1]
Phase Contrast MRA(相位对比MRA)	Phase-contrast MRA (PC MRA) is a gradient echo sequence that depicts blood flow by quantifying differences in the transverse magnetization between stationary and moving tissue [1]
Physical biomarkers of stroke(脑卒中的物理生物标志物)	A physical marker associated with stroke may be as simple as the discovery of hypertension [1]
Physical Examination(查体)	An observation of the body or a body part using one of the five human senses (e.g. inspection, palpation, percussion, auscultation) An observation of the body or a body part using one of the five human senses (e.g., inspection, palpation, percussion, auscultation) [1]
Physical therapy(理疗)	又称"物理疗法"。应用力、电、光、声、磁、冷、热、水等方法对疾病进行预防、治疗和康复的方法。是物理医学与康复的一个重要组成部分。通常分运动疗法和物理因子疗法[3]

续　表

英文术语（中文术语）	定义（英文和/或中文）
Platelet factor 4(血小板因子4)	A CXC chemokine that is found in the alpha granules of PLATELETS. The protein has a molecular size of 7800 kDa and can occur as a monomer, a dimer or a tetramer depending upon its concentration in solution. Platelet factor 4 has a high affinity for HEPARIN and is often found complexed with GLYCOPROTEINS such as PROTEIN C[1]
Poly ADP ribose polymerase activation(多聚ADP核糖聚合酶活化)	PADP is a mediators facilitate apoptotic cell death pathways[1]
Polyamine metabolites(多胺类代谢产物)	Polyamines complex with RNA and facilitate translation. The polyamine spermine has been evaluated in acute stroke, together with spermine oxidase (SMO) and acetylpolyamine oxidase (AcPAO), enzymes that catalyze its degradation, and proteinconjugated acrolein, one of its metabolites[1]
Pontine infarct symptom(桥脑梗死症状)	Pontine infarcts are one form of brainstem infarction involving the posterior circulation. Infarcts in the pons are typically focal in nature[1]
Post stroke dementia(卒中后痴呆)	Poststroke dementia (PSD) is one of the main causes of dependency in survivors and includes any dementia after a stroke, irrespective of its cause—ie, vascular, degenerative, or mixed[1]
Post stroke depression(卒中后抑郁)	Depression is a common complication post-stroke affecting approximately one-third of patients. The presence of post-stroke depression has been associated with decreases in functional recovery, social activity and cognition[1]
Posterior cerebral artery infarction syndrome (大脑后动脉梗死综合征)	The PCA is subdivided into four segments with associated clinical presentation. An occlusion of the proximal segment (P1 or precommunal) usually causes a total PCA infarction, including upper midbrain, variable parts of the thalamus and posterior hemispheric territory. Occlusions of the P2 (or postcommunal) segment before the branching of the thalamogeniculate arteries provoke ischemic lesions in the lateral thalamus and the hemispheric PCA territory. Lastly, cortical PCA branch occlusion causes diverse cortical lesions in the superficial PCA territory, including the occipital, postero-inferior temporal and variable part of the posterior parietal lobes[1]

英文术语（中文术语）	定义（英文和/或中文）
Posterior Choroidal artery infarction symptom(脉络膜后动脉梗死症状)	The PChA arising from the P2 segment of the PCA, and is subdivided into medial and lateral branches. They supply the pulvinar, part of the lateral and medial geniculate body, the posterior parts of the intralaminar nuclei, and lateral dorsal and lateral posterior nuclei. They also irrigate posterior portions of medial temporal structures, parts of midbrain and probably the subthalamic nucleus[1]
Postural Assessment Scale for Stroke Patients(脑卒中患者体位评估量表)	The Postural Assessment Scale for Stroke patients (PASS), adapted from the BL Motor Assessment, was elaborated in concordance with 3 main ideas: (1) the ability to maintain a given posture and to ensure equilibrium in changing position both must be assessed; (2) the scale should be applicable for all patients, even those with very poor postural performance; and (3) it should contain items with increasing difficulty. The PASS is one of the most valid and reliable clinical assessments of postural control in stroke patients during the first 3 months after stroke[1]
Postural tremor(姿势性震颤)	A type of tremors that is triggered by holding a limb in a fixed position[2]
Postural tremor(姿势性震颤)	当固定肢体在一个位置时诱发的震颤[2]
pressure sore rehabilitation nursing(压疮康复护理)	护理工作者对卧床的患者采取定时翻身、骨凸起部位皮肤的减压及清洁，防治皮肤破溃的护理方法[3]
Primary stroke center(初级卒中中心)	A PSC has the personnel, programs, expertise, and infrastructure to care for many patients with uncomplicated strokes, uses many acute therapies (such as intravenous rtPA), and admits such patients into a stroke unit[1]
Prior stroke(既往卒中)	prior stroke is a strong predisposing risk factor for new stroke and is the most common disease with ICH[1]
Processed meat(加工肉制品)	Consumption of processed meat is associated with an increased risk of stroke[1]
Progressive gait ataxia(进行性共济失调)	A type of "gait ataxia" (HP:0002066) displaying progression of clinical severity[2]
Progressive gait ataxia(进行性共济失调)	随着临床病程的推移而进行性加重的共济失调[2]
Progressive ptosis(进行性上睑下垂)	A "progressive" (PATO:0001818) form of "ptosis" (HP:0000508)[2]

续　表

英文术语（中文术语）	定义（英文和/或中文）
Progressive ptosis(进行性上睑下垂)	上睑下垂逐渐加重[2]
Progressive visual field defects(进行性视野缺损)	visual field defects Progressively[2]
Progressive visual field defects(进行性视野缺损)	进行性发生的视野缺损[2]
Projectile vomiting(喷射性呕吐)	Vomiting that ejects the gastric contents with great force[2]
Projectile vomiting(喷射性呕吐)	胃内容物以很大力量喷射性呕吐出来[2]
Prosopagnosia(面容失认)	Prosopagnosia denotes the inability to recognize previously known faces, whereas voice recognition remains normal and allows the patients to compensate their deficit in everyday life[1]
Protanomaly(红色弱视)	A type of anomalous trichromacy associated with defective long-wavelength-sensitive (L) cones, causing the sensitivity spectrum to be shifted toward medium wavelengths. This leads to difficulties especially in distinguishing red and green[2]
Protanomaly(红色弱视)	三色视中感受长光波红光的视锥细胞缺陷，导致光谱敏感性向中等长度光方向移动，导致红色和绿色分辨困难[2]
Protanopia(红色盲)	Blue and green cones only; no functional red cones[2]
Protanopia(红色盲)	只有蓝色和绿色锥体；无功能性红色视锥细胞[2]
Proton magnetic resonance spectroscopy image(质子磁共振波谱图像)	Proton magnetic resonance spectroscopic imaging (H-MRS) and diffusion weighted imaging have been used to measure the cerebral lactate and N-acetylaspartate (NAA) levels in acute cerebral ischemia[1]
prudent diet(谨慎饮食)	A prudent diet, characterised by high intakes of fruits, vegetables, legumes, fi sh, and whole grains, was associated with a lower risk of stroke after 14 years of follow-up of 71 768 women (relative risk 0•78, 95% CI 0•61–1•01; comparing extreme quintiles) whereas a western diet, characterised by high intakes of red and processed meats, refi ned grains, and sweets and desserts, was associated with an increased risk of stroke (relative risk 1•58, 95% CI 1•15–2•15; comparing the highest with lowest quintiles of the western diet)[1]

英文术语（中文术语）	定义（英文和/或中文）
Pseudobulbar palsy(假性球麻痹)	Bilateral impairment of the function of the cranial nerves 9-12, which control musculature involved in eating, swallowing, and speech. Pseudobulbar paralysis is characterized clinically by dysarthria, dysphonia, and dysphagia with bifacial paralysis, and may be accompanied by "Pseudobulbar behavioral symptoms" (HP:0002193) such as enforced crying and laughing[2]
Pseudobulbar palsy(假性球麻痹)	第9-12对颅神经控制与进食、吞咽、讲话相关的肌肉，双侧受损时表现为假性球麻痹。假性球麻痹以构音障碍、发音困难、吞咽困难伴双侧面瘫为临床特征，可能伴有强哭强笑等"假性球麻痹性行为症状"[2]
Pseudoradicular sensory deficit(假性神经根感觉障碍)	Sensory impairments may be found in the affected half of the body, particularly in the lower limb, although usually they are mild or indefinite, or sometimes totally absent. The modalities most often involved are discriminative and proprioceptive[1]
Pseudoseizure with tonic spasm(假性发作伴强直性痉挛)	Pseudoseizure is characterized by paroxysmal behavioral alterations that may resemble epileptic seizures. Impaired responsiveness to external or internal stimuli (or both) and involuntary movements, often dramatic, are common features. seudoseizures are often a conversion symptom ("hysterical seizures") and may coexist with other neurologic or nonneurologic illnesses[1]
Ptosis(上睑下垂)	The upper eyelid margin is positioned 3 mm or more lower than usual and covers the superior portion of the iris (objective); or, the upper lid margin obscures at least part of the pupil (subjective)[2]
Ptosis(上睑下垂)	上睑缘比正常位置低3毫米或更多，覆盖虹膜的上部分（客观角度）;或者遮蔽一部分进入瞳孔的光线（主观角度）[2]
Pulmonary embolism(肺栓塞)	Pulmonary embolism is an obstruction of a blood vessel in the lungs, usually due to a blood clot, which blocks a coronary artery[1]

续　表

英文术语（中文术语）	定义（英文和/或中文）
Pulsatile tinnitus(搏动性耳鸣)	Pulsatile tinnitus is generally classified a kind of objective tinnitus, meaning that it is not only audible to the patient but also to the examiner on auscultation of the auditory canal and/or of surrounding structures with use of an auscultation tube or stethoscope. Usually, pulsatile tinnitus is heard as a lower pitched thumping or booming, a rougher blowing sound which is coincidental with respiration, or as a clicking, higher pitched rhythmic sensation. Pulsatile tinnitus may be associated with vascular abnormalities such as arterioevenous shunts or glomus tumors or the jugular vein, arterial bruits related to a high-riding carotid artery (close to the auditory areas) or carotid stenosis, or venous abnormalities such as a dehiscent jugular bulb or to hypertension. Finally, in some patients, mechanical abnormalities such a spatulous eustachian tubes, palatomyoclonus (small spasms of muscles in the soft palate area), or idiopathic stapedial muscle spasm may represent the underlying cause of pulsatile tinnitus[2]
Pulsatile tinnitus(搏动性耳鸣)	搏动性耳鸣通常被分类为客观性耳鸣，意味着不仅是病人可听及耳鸣声音，检查者应用听诊管或听诊器对耳道和/或其周围结构进行听诊时亦可听及。搏动性耳鸣一般为低的重击声或者隆隆声，粗糙的与呼吸一致的吹风声，或者为较高音调的有节奏感的敲击声。搏动性耳鸣可能与血管异常相关，如动静脉分流、颈静脉球体瘤，高位颈动脉（近听觉区域）相关的动脉杂音或颈动脉狭窄，或静脉异常如颈静脉球开裂或高血压。最后，在一些患者中，机械异常如咽鼓管扩张、腭肌阵挛（软腭区域肌肉小痉挛）或特发性镫骨肌痉挛也可能是搏动性耳鸣的根本原因[2]
Pure motor hemiparesis(纯运动性轻偏瘫)	Pure motor hemiparesis (PMH) was reported by Fisher and Curry (1965) as an acute pure motor stroke involving face, arm, and leg on one side, in the absence of sensory deficit, homonymous hemianopia, aphasia, agnosia, or apraxia[1]
Pure sensory stroke(纯感觉性卒中)	Pure sensory stroke is usually related to a lesion in the ventroposterior nucleus of the thalamus, and less frequently the corona radiata[1]

英文术语（中文术语）	定义（英文和/或中文）
push method(推举法)	增加软腭肌肌力的言语训练方法。将患者双手放在桌面上向下推；两手掌由下向上推；两手掌相对推或两手掌同时向下推同时发[au]的声音[3]
Raymond syndrome(Raymond综合征)	Raymond syndrome is characterised by ipsilateral abducens nerve palsy and contralateral hemiplegia[1]
Reactive oxygen species generation(活性氧生成)	Reactive oxygen species [ROS] have been implicated in brain injury after ischemic stroke. There is evidence that a rapid increase in the production of ROS immediately after acute ischemic stroke rapidly overwhelm antioxidant defences, causing further tissue damage. These ROS can damage cellular macromolecules leading to autophagy, apoptosis, and necrosis. Moreover, the rapid restoration of blood flow increases the level of tissue oxygenation and accountsfor a second burst of ROS generation, which leads to reperfusion injury[1]
Red meat intake(红肉摄入量)	Higher intake of red meat (1 serving/day) was associated with an elevated risk of stroke[1]
Red-green dyschromatopsia(红绿色觉障碍)	Difficulty with discriminating red and green hues[2]
Red-green dyschromatopsia(红绿色觉障碍)	识别红色和绿色色调困难[2]
Reduced fat milk(低脂牛奶)	Reduced-fat milk (vs full-strength milk) Consumption is associated with lower risk of stroke[1]
Rehabilitation nursing of hemiplegia(偏瘫康复护理)	对偏瘫患者采取心肺护理、大小便护理、皮肤护理、良肢位摆放、翻身方法等措施。预防偏瘫患者出现并发症和合并症[3]
Resting tremor(静止性震颤)	A resting tremor occurs when muscles are at rest and becomes less noticeable or disappears when the affected muscles are moved. Resting tremors are often slow and coarse[2]
Resting tremor(静止性震颤)	静止性震颤发生在肌肉静息时，当受累肌肉活动时变得很轻或消失，是缓慢的、粗大的震颤[2]
Retinol(视黄醇)	Retinol and derivatives of retinol that play an essential role in metabolic functioning of the retina, the growth of and differentiation of epithelial tissue, the growth of bone, reproduction, and the immune response. Dietary vitamin A is derived from a variety of CAROTENOIDS found in plants. It is enriched in the liver, egg yolks, and the fat component of dairy products[1]

续　表

英文术语（中文术语）	定义（英文和/或中文）
Retrocollis(颈后倾)	A form of "torticollis" (HP:0000473) in which the head is drawn back, either due to a permanent contractures of neck extensor muscles, or to a spasmodic contracture [2]
Retrocollis(颈后倾)	由于颈部伸肌持续性性或阵发性挛缩导致头部向后倾斜 [2]
Rice intake(大米摄入量)	Rice consumption has been associated with an increased risk of stroke [1]
Ring scotoma(环形暗点)	Ring scotoma [2]
Ring scotoma(环形暗点)	环形的暗点 [2]
Risk factor(危险因素)	An aspect of personal behavior or lifestyle, environmental exposure, or inborn or inherited characteristic, which, on the basis of epidemiologic evidence, is known to be associated with a health-related condition considered important to prevent [1]
Risk factor reduction(降低风险因素)	Risk-reduction measures in primary stroke prevention may include the use of antihypertensive medications; warfarin; platelet antiaggregants; 3-hydroxy-3-methylglutaryl coenzyme A (HMG-CoA) reductase inhibitors (statins); smoking cessation; dietary intervention; weight loss; and exercise. Modifiable risk factors include the following: Hypertension, Cigarette smoking, Diabetes, Dyslipidemiam, Atrial fibrillation, Sickle cell disease, Postmenopausal HRT, Depression, Diet and activity, Weight and body fat [1]
Rivaroxaban(利伐沙班)	Rivaroxaban is an orally active, direct-acting Factor Xa inhibitor with bioavailability of more than 80% [1]
Rivermead Behavioral Inattention Test (Rivermead行为注意力测试)	The Rivermead Behavioral Inattention Test (RBIT), consisting of nine items sampling activities of daily living, [1]
Rivermead Mobility Index(Rivermead活动指数)	The Rivermead Mobility Index (RMI) is a hierarchical mobility scale used in neurological rehabilitation. It includes 15 items related to bed mobility, transfers, walking, stair use, and running. The RMI is presented in a questionnaire format with the examiner required to make one observation (standing unsupported >10 s). All items are rated in a yes/no format with positive responses scoring a 1 for a maximal RMI score of 15 [1]

英文术语（中文术语）	定义（英文和/或中文）
Rotary nystagmus(旋转性眼球震颤)	A form of nystagmus in which the eyeball makes rotary motions around the axis[2]
Rotary nystagmus(旋转性眼球震颤)	眼球震颤的一种形式，眼球绕轴旋转[2]
rt-PA(阿替普酶)	Alteplase is a t-PA used in management of acute myocardial infarction (MI), acute ischemic stroke, and pulmonary embolism. Safety and efficacy with concomitant administration of heparin or aspirin during the first 24 hours after symptom onset have not been investigated[1]
Rubral tremor(红核震颤)	Rubral tremor is characterized by a slow coarse tremor at rest that is exacerbated by postural adjustments and by guided voluntary movements[2]
Rubral tremor(红核震颤)	红核震颤的特征是休息时缓慢的粗糙震颤，姿势调整和自主运动会导致震颤加剧[2]
S100 beta(S100β)	S100-beta (S100B) is a calcium-binding peptide secreted by astrocytes in the context of brain injury, neurodegenerative processes and psychiatric disorders[1]
SATIS Stroke(SATIS卒中)	Satis-Stroke is a satisfaction measure of activities and participation in the actual environment experienced by patients after chronic stroke using the Rasch measurement model[1]
Scales(量表)	Stroke scales are useful for clinical and research purposes as aids to improve diagnostic accuracy, determine the suitability of specific treatments, monitor change in neurologic impairments, and predict and measure outcomes[1]
Scandinavian stroke scale(斯堪得维亚脑卒中量表)	The scandinavian stroke scale was developed to test therapeutic efficacy of hemodilution treatment in acute middle cerebral artery stroke[1]
scapula mobilization(肩胛骨松动术)	用以维持肩胸关节正常活动度，以便偏瘫侧上肢能全关节活动范围运动而免于产生肩关节疼痛和活动受限，且抑制上肢屈肌痉挛的一种治疗技术。操作可在仰卧位、侧卧位和坐位下进行[3]
Scavenger Receptors, Class A(清道夫受体，A类)	A family of scavenger receptors that mediate the influx of LIPIDS into MACROPHAGES and are involved in FOAM CELL formation[1]

续　表

英文术语（中文术语）	定义（英文和/或中文）
Schuellapha-sic stimulation approach(许尔失语症刺激疗法)	对损害的语言符号系统应用强的、控制下的听觉刺激为基础，最大程度地促进失语症患者的语言再建和恢复的失语症训练方法。是多种失语症治疗方法的基础[3]
Scintillating scotoma(闪光性暗点)	A scintillating scotoma is a common visual aura that can preced a migraine, whereby a spot of flickering light near the center of the visual fields occurs. The spot prevents vision, and is thus termed scotoma. The scotoma can extend into one or more shimmering arcs of white or colored flashing lights[2]
Scintillating scotoma(闪光性暗点)	闪烁的暗点是一种常见的视觉先兆，可以是偏头痛的先兆，其中闪烁的灯光在视野中心点附近出现。盲点可延伸进入白色或有色闪灯的一个或多个波光弧[2]
Scotoma(暗点)	Scotoma refers to an area or island of loss or impairment of visual acuity surrounded by a field of normal or relatively well-preserved vision[2]
Scotoma(暗点)	盲点是指一个区域视觉敏锐度受损，这一区域被正常或相对完好的视力范围包饶[2]
Screening for diabetic mellitus(糖尿病筛查)	After a TIA or ischemic stroke, all patients should probably be screened for DM with testing of fasting plasma glucose, HbA1c, or an oral glucose tolerance test[1]
Screening for Self Medication Safety Post Stroke Scale(脑卒中后自我用药安全量表筛查)	The Screening for Safe Self-medication post-Stroke Scale (S-5) has been created and validated for use by health professionals to screen self-medication safety readiness of patients after stroke. Its use should also help to guide clinicians' recommendations and interventions aimed at enhancing self-medication post-stroke[1]
Seesaw nystagmus(跷跷板眼球震颤)	Seesaw nystagmus is a type of pendular nystagmus where a half cycle consists of the elevation and intorsion of one eye, concurrently with the depression and extortion of the fellow eye. In the other half cycle, there is an inversion of the ocular movements[2]
Seesaw nystagmus(跷跷板眼球震颤)	跷跷板眼球震颤是一种摆动眼球震颤，其中一半周期表现为一只眼睛的升高和内旋，同时另一只眼睛下降和外展。在另一半周期中，眼运动反转[2]
Sensorimotor stroke(感觉运动性卒中)	Sensorimotor stroke may result from a lesion of the internal capsule, and rarely from the paramedian pons[1]

英文术语（中文术语）	定义（英文和/或中文）
Serum albumin(白蛋白)	Albumin itself shows a neuroprotective effect in animal models of ischemic stroke. It was suggested that this neuroprotective effect was mediated by multiple specific actions of albumin, including antioxidative properties, and influence on endothelial functions and venular perfusion[1]
serum lipid test(血脂检测)	Serum lipid profile is measured for cardiovascular risk prediction and has now become almost a routine test. The test includes four basic parameters: total cholesterol, HDL cholesterol, LDL cholesterol and triglycerides[1]
Shoulder pain(肩痛)	Unilateral or bilateral pain of the shoulder. It is often caused by physical activities such as work or sports participation, but may also be pathologic in origin[1]
Shwartz Index(史华兹指数)	The Shwartz Index consists of 21 weighted conditions and evaluates the negative influence of comorbid conditions on the treatment of the primary condition, including stroke, lung disease, heart disease, prostate disease, low back disorders, and hip fracture[1]
Sickle cell disease(镰状细胞血症)	Sickle-cell disease is one of the most important hemoglobinopathies and the most prevalent form of congenital hemolytic anemia[1]
Simultanagnosia(综合性失认)	Simultagnosia typically occurs in the absence of visual field deficits. Although the ability to perceive and name individual objects regardless of their location within the visual field remains intact, patients with simultagnosia exhibit an inability to perceive and interpret the overall gestalt of the scene. Simultagnosia usually results from bilateral lesions to the parietal-occipital regions, though some cases have been reported following damage to the superior occipital or inferior parietal lobes[1]
Six Minute Walk Test(六分钟步行测试)	The six-minute walk test (6MWT) measures the distance (6MWD) that a person can quickly walk on a flat, hard surface in 6 min. The test is submaximal and self-paced, with rest breaks allowed as needed[1]
Skew deviation(反向偏斜)	ocular divergence in the vertical plane[1]
Sleep myoclonus(睡眠肌阵挛)	Myoclonus that occurs during the initial phases of sleep[2]

续　表

英文术语（中文术语）	定义（英文和/或中文）
Sleep myoclonus(睡眠肌阵挛)	在睡眠的初始阶段出现的肌阵挛[2]
Smoking cessation(戒烟)	Cigarette smoking is an independent risk factor for ischemic stroke, and growing evidence has shown that exposure to environmental smoke increases the risk of cardiovascular disease, including stroke. Smoking cessation is recommended in persons who have experienced a stroke or TIA[1]
Soda intake(苏打摄入量)	Greater consumption of sugar-sweetened and low-calorie sodas was associated with a significantly higher risk of stroke[1]
Sodium intake(钠盐摄入)	A higher sodium intake is associated with an increased risk of stroke; The recommended sodium intake is <2.3 g/d (100 mmol/d)[1]
Somnolence(嗜睡状态)	omnolence (alternatively "sleepiness" or "drowsiness") is a state of strong desire for sleep, or sleeping for unusually long periods (compare hypersomnia)[1]
Spasmus nutans(点头痉挛)	The combination of pendular nystagmus, head nodding, and torticollis[2]
Spastic dysarthria(痉挛性构音障碍)	A type of dysarthria related to bilateral damage of the upper motor neuron tracts of the pyramidal and extra- pyramidal tracts. Speech of affected individuals is slow, effortful, and has a harsh vocal quality[2]
Spastic dysarthria(痉挛性构音障碍)	一种与双侧上运动神经元的锥体束和锥体外束损伤相关的构音障碍。受累的个体的语言缓慢、费力而且音质刺耳[2]
Speech apraxia(失读症)	A type of apraxia that is characterized by difficulty or inability to execute speech movements because of problems with coordination and motor problems, leading to incorrect articulation. An increase of errors with increasing word and phrase length may occur[2]
Speech apraxia(失读症)	是一种失用的，其特征因为协调和运动问题导致执行语言运动困难或不能，从而导致不正确发音。随着单词和短语的长度的增加发生的错误的可能性也会增加[2]
Spermine oxidase(精胺氧化酶)	A protein that is a translation product of the human SMOX gene or a 1:1 ortholog thereof[1]
Sphincter of Oddi dysfunction(Oddi括约肌功能障碍)	the sphincter muscle does not open when it should[1]

英文术语（中文术语）	定义（英文和/或中文）
Spinal myoclonus(脊髓肌阵挛)	Spinal myoclonus is generally due to a tumor, infection, injury, or degenerative process of the spinal cord, and is characterized by involuntary rhythmic muscle contractions, usually at a rate of more than one per second. Myoclonus occurs synchronously in several muscles and can be increased in severity and frequency by fatigue or stress, but is usually unaffected by sensory stimuli. Spinal myoclonus ceases during sleep or anesthesia[2]
Spinal myoclonus(脊髓肌阵挛)	脊肌阵挛通常是由于一个肿瘤、感染、损伤，或脊髓变性过程，其特征是节律不自主的肌肉收缩，通常在一个以上的每秒的速率。同步发生肌阵挛在几个肌肉和所用的严重程度和频率由疲劳或应力增加，但通常是不受感官刺激。睡眠或麻醉期间脊髓性肌阵挛停止[2]
sport(运动)	For patients with ischemic stroke or TIA who are capable of engaging in physical activity, at least 3 to 4 sessions per week of moderate- to vigorous-intensity aerobic physical exercise are reasonable to reduce stroke risk factors. Sessions should last an average of 40 minutes[1]
Stay away from alcoholic drinks(戒酒)	Moderate alcohol consumption[1]
Stop Stroke Study TOAST(改良TOAST分型)	The SSS-TOAST is composed of the same five major stroke subtypes in the TOAST classification system. In the SSS-TOAST system, each causative category is subdivided based on the weight of evidence as "evident" "probable," or "possible"[1]
Stroke Activity Scale(脑卒中活动量表)	The Stroke Activity Scale (SAS) assesses activities of daily living beyond the limited self-care assessments previously available. The author'sgoal was to develop a brief scale of lifestyle to determine rehabilitation goals. The SAS is a five-item scale that was developed by physiotherapists as a measure of motor function at the level of disability in stroke patients for use in the clinical setting. It consists of five items (getting out of bed, sitting balance, sitting to standing, stepping and walking, and bringing a glass to the mouth) that take fewer than 10 min to administer[1]

续　表

英文术语（中文术语）	定义（英文和/或中文）
Stroke Adapted Sickness Impact Profile(卒中适应疾病影响分布)	An adaptation of the full version of the 136-item Sickness Impact Profile (SIP). The Stroke-Adapted Sickness Impact Profile (SA-SIP30) contains 30 items within 8 subscales: body care and movement, social interaction, mobility, communication, emotional behavior, household management, alertness behavior, and ambulation. Scoring for the SA-SIP30 is conducted in the same manner as for the full version SIP and yields the same subscales, dimensions, and total score. Total scores range from 0% to 100% with higher scores corresponding to worse health[1]
Stroke Aphasic Depression Questionnaire (脑卒中双相抑郁问卷)	The Stroke Aphasic Depression Questionnaire was developed by Sutcliffe and Lincoln (1998) to assess mood in aphasic stroke patients and to monitor patients progress with treatment[1]
Stroke Arm Ladder(卒中臂梯)	The goal of this measure is to parsimoniously quantify upper extremity function after stroke through a tailored "test" made up of items suited to their level of upper extremity function[1]
Stroke Impact Scale(脑卒中影响量表)	The Stroke Impact Scale (SIS) is a quality of life measure designed specifically for patients with stroke. The instrument is a self-report questionnaire assessing eight domains: strength, hand function, activities of daily living (ADL)/instrumental ADL (IADL), mobility, communication, emotion, memory and thinking, and social participation. Each item is rated on a scale from 1 to 5 (indicating either high or low quality of life, depending on the specific question) and an additional item assesses the patient's global perception of percent recovery[1]
Stroke recurrence(卒中复发)	Recurrent stroke is frequent and responsible for major stroke morbidity and mortality[1]
Stroke Specific Quality Of Life scale(卒中特异性生活质量量表)	The SS-QOL is a single stroke outcome measure that aims to efficiently assess the various domains important in determining stroke-specific HRQOL across the spectrum of stroke symptoms and severity[1]

英文术语（中文术语）	定义（英文和/或中文）
Stupor(昏睡)	Stupor correspond to more advanced stages of impaired arousal. In stupor patients usually appear to be asleep and awaken only when stimulated with a loud voice or vigorous shaking. They may be agitated or combative at such times but they do not communicate in a meaningful way apart from monosyllabic sounds, groans, and simple behaviors. They return to a sleep-like state as soon as stimulation ceases[1]
Subdural hemorrhage(硬膜下出血)	ccumulation of blood in the SUBDURAL SPACE between the DURA MATER and the arachnoidal layer of the MENINGES. This condition primarily occurs over the surface of a CEREBRAL HEMISPHERE, but may develop in the spinal canal (HEMATOMA, SUBDURAL, SPINAL). Subdural hematoma can be classified as the acute or the chronic form, with immediate or delayed symptom onset, respectively. Symptoms may include loss of consciousness, severe HEADACHE, and deteriorating mental status[1]
Subsequent herniation(继发脑疝)	Because the intracranial compartments are generally noncompressible and the intracranial volume is essentially constant, any additional pressure-producing solid or liquid mass within the intracranial cavity will result in displacement of healthy tissues. Supratentorial expanding mass lesions, such as tumors, abscesses, ischemic or hemorrhagic strokes, or traumatic hematomas, can produce herniation by displacing adjacent and remote brain tissue, especially diencephalon. Such displacement may occur across the midline (e.g., subfalcian herniation) or via the rostro-caudal direction by compressing the deep diencephalic and midbrain structures (e.g., uncal and central herniation)[1]
Superior cerebellar artery infarction symptom (小脑上动脉梗死症状)	An isolated SCA syndrome is rare, but the territory is regularly involved in distal basilar artery occlusion[1]
Superoxide radicals(超氧化物)	superoxide (O2) is an oxygen molecule deficient of on electron. superoxide radicals are formed normally in the body and may involved in the regulation of fibroblast proliferation, vasodilatation and phagocytosis[1]

续　表

英文术语（中文术语）	定义（英文和/或中文）
Syncope(晕厥)	Syncope is defined as a short and transient loss of consciousness with loss of postural control. Syncope is rarely caused by TIA or stroke. Among a series of 551 patients with acute cerebrovascular disorders, syncope was observed in 6% of those who had suffered stroke and in less than 1% of those with TIAs, more often in the carotid than in the vertebrobasilar territory. About half of all cases were attributed to seizures, and the rest to brainstem ischemia (with impairment of the ARAS) or to bihemispheric dysfunction related to diaschisis[1]
Syncope(晕厥)	Syncope is defined as a short loss of consciousness and muscle strength, characterized by a fast onset, short duration, and spontaneous recovery[2]
Syncope(晕厥)	晕厥是指暂时性意识丧失和肌肉无力，特点是发作迅速，持续时间短，能自然恢复[2]
Tau protein(Tau蛋白)	Tau protein (TP) is a structural microtubule-associated protein that is well known for its association with a variety of neurodegenerative disorders, including Alzheimer's disease[1]
Tea intake(茶摄入量)	the consumption of tea (>3 cups) has been associated with a reduction in the risk of stroke[1]
Tecarfarin(特卡法林)	Tecarfarin (ATI-5923) is a novel oral vitamin K antagonist. Unlike warfarin, it is metabolized by esterases, escaping metabolism by the cytochrome P450 system and thereby avoiding cytochrome P450-mediated drug-drug or drug-food interactions as well as genetic variations found in the cytochrome P450 system[1]
Telemedicine(远程医疗)	Delivery of health services via remote telecommunications. This includes interactive consultative and diagnostic services. Health services supported by remote or mobile devices[1]
telemetry technology(遥测技术)	Transmission of the readings of instruments to a remote location by means of wires, radio waves, or other means. (McGraw-Hill Dictionary of Scientific and Technical Terms, 4th ed)[1]

英文术语（中文术语）	定义（英文和/或中文）
Temporospatial disorientation(时空定向障碍)	Disorientation is an alteration of mental status characterized by lack of awareness of personal identity, place, time, and/or situation. Typically, disorientation occurs first in time, then in place, and finally in person. It is assessed by asking the person specific questions in these spheres. Disorientation is a relatively nonspecific symptom occurring in diffuse disorders (i.e., dementia), focal brain lesions (i.e., stroke), and infectious and metabolic processes; secondary to medications and drug interactions; and in psychological disorders (i.e., schizophrenia)[1]
Tension-type headache(紧张性头痛)	A type of headache that last hours with continuous pain of mild or moderate intensity, bilateral location, a pressing/tightening (non-pulsating) quality and that is not aggravated by routine physical activity such as walking or climbing stairs[2]
Tension-type headache(紧张性头痛)	是一种持续数小时的持续性轻到中度的双侧性头痛，性质为压迫性或紧缩性（非搏动性）并且日常体力活动如行走、爬楼梯不会加重[2]
Tetracycline antibiotics(四环素类抗生素)	The tetracycline family of antibiotics has also been shown to reduce leukocyte infiltration and improve experimental stroke outcome[1]
Tetraparesis(四肢轻瘫)	Tetraplegia refers to a complete loss of strength, whereas Tetraparesis refers to an incomplete loss of strength. Weakness of all four limbs[1]
Tetraplegia(四肢瘫)	Paralysis of all four limbs, and trunk of the body below the level of an associated injury to the spinal cord. The etiology of quadriplegia is similar to that of paraplegia except that the lesion is in the cervical spinal cord rather than in the thoracic or lumbar segments of the spinal cord[2]
Tetraplegia(四肢瘫)	相关的脊髓损伤水平以下的所有四肢、躯干的麻痹。四肢瘫的病因是类似于截瘫的不同之处在于病变是在颈脊髓而不是在脊髓的胸腰椎段[2]
Thalamic aphasia(丘脑性失语)	Aphasia can also follow thalamic hemorrhages or infarcts of the dominant hemisphere. The first reports of thalamic hemorrhages causing aphasia stressed the decreased voice volume, anomia, perseveration, and semantic paraphasia[1]

225

续　表

英文术语（中文术语）	定义（英文和/或中文）
Thalamic dementia(丘脑性痴呆)	Cognitive disturbances consist mostly of personality changes with disinhibited behavior, impulsivity, apathy and even loss of psychic selfactivation associated with amnesia similar to Korsakoff syndrome. This picture of amnesia and behavioral disturbances is recognized as a "thalamic dementia"[1]
Thalamic infarction syndrome(丘脑梗死综合征)	The thalamus is a centrally situated structure with extensive reciprocal connections with the cortex, basal ganglia and brainstem nuclei. Therefore it can mimic cortical and subcortical strokes in the anterior or posterior circulation and is also called "the great imitator". Its vascularization is subdivided into four territories correlated with the organization of the thalamic nuclei: - the tuberothalamic (or polar) artery -the thalamogeniculate (or inferolateral) artery -the paramedian arteries -the posterior choroidal artery (PChA)[1]
Thalamic pain syndrom(丘脑痛综合征)	Contralateral loss of or diminished somatosensory sensation, particularly proprioception or position sense following a thalamic lesion. The syndrome most commonly results from a vascular lesion affecting the ventral posterior nucleus. Most notable in this syndrome is the concomitant presence of diffuse, lingering pain which may be produced by relatively minor and even noncutaneous stimuli, while the response to actual painful-type stimuli may be diminished[1]
Thalamogeniculate artery infarction symptom(丘脑膝状体动脉梗死症状)	The thalamogeniculate (or inferolateral) arteries are a group of 5–10 arteries arising from the P2 segment of the PCA. The principal branches supply the ventrolateral nucleus and the ventroposterior nuclei, while the medial branches supply the medial geniculate body and the inferior branches the rostral and lateral pulvinar, as well as the laterodorsal nucleus[1]
THAM(三羟甲基氨基甲烷)	THAM is supposed to act by entering the cerebrospinal fluid compartment and neutralizing the acidosis-induced vasodilation, thereby reducing ICP. ICP-lowering properties as well as beneficial effects on edema formation and cerebral energy disturbance of THAM have been demonstrated in animal models of head injury. In animal models of focal cerebral ischemia, THAM infusion was associated with a significant reduction of infarct size, brain edema and lactate concentration[1]

英文术语（中文术语）	定义（英文和/或中文）
Thiobarbituric acid reactive substances(硫代巴比妥酸反应物质)	Low-molecular-weight end products, probably malondialdehyde, that are formed during the decomposition of lipid peroxidation products. These compounds react with thiobarbituric acid to form a fluorescent red adduct [1]
Thrombin activable fibrinolysis inhibitor(凝血酶活性纤溶抑制剂)	A protein that is a translation product of the human CPB2 gene or a 1∶1 ortholog thereof. Category=gene [1]
thromboembolism(血栓栓塞)	An "embolism" is a blood clot that forms in one part of the body and then travels (or embolizes) to another area in the body, and an embolic stroke is one in which a blood clot travels from one place in the body to another [1]
Thrombolysis in cerebral infarction(脑梗死时溶栓)	The thrombolysis in cerebral infarction (TICI) grading system was described in 2003 by Higashida et al as a tool for determining the response of thrombolytic therapy for ischaemic stroke. In neurointerventional radiology it is usually used for patients post endovascular revascularisation. Like most therapy response grading systems, it predicts prognosis [1]
Thrombomodulin(血栓调节蛋白)	Thrombomodulin (TM) is an endothelial membrane protein that plays an important role in hemostasis by binding thrombin and activating protein C, thereby exerting an antithrombotic mechanism [1]
Thrombophilia(易栓症)	Hypercoagulable states are another unusual cause of stroke. There is a constant interplay in the body between factors that cause the blood to clot, or coagulate, and factors that cause the blood to remain liquid [1]
Thrombosis(血栓形成)	Thrombosis is a critical event in the arterial diseases associated with myocardial infarction and stroke, and venous thromboembolic disorders account for considerable morbidity and mortality [1]
Thunderclap headache(霹雳样头痛)	Severe head pain with sudden onset, reaching its maximum intensity in less than one minute and lasting from one hour to ten days [2]
Thunderclap headache(霹雳样头痛)	严重头痛突然发作，在不到一分钟内达到最大强度，持续1小时至10天 [2]

续　表

英文术语（中文术语）	定义（英文和/或中文）
Tinnitus(耳鸣)	Tinnitus is an auditory perception that can be described as the experience of sound, in the ear or in the head, in the absence of external acoustic stimulation[2]
Tinnitus(耳鸣)	耳鸣是一种没有外部声刺激却出现声音相关的听觉体验，这种体验常位于耳朵或头颅中[2]
Tissue inhibitors of metalloproteinase 1(基质金属蛋白酶抑制剂1)	A member of the family of TISSUE INHIBITOR OF METALLOPROTEINASES. It is a N-glycosylated protein, molecular weight 28 kD, produced by a vast range of cell types and found in a variety of tissues and body fluids. It has been shown to suppress metastasis and inhibit tumor invasion in vitro[1]
Tissue inhibitors of metalloproteinase 2(基质金属蛋白酶抑制剂2)	A member of the family of TISSUE INHIBITOR OF METALLOPROTEINASES. It is a 21-kDa nonglycosylated protein found in tissue fluid and is secreted as a complex with progelatinase A by human fibroblast and uncomplexed from alveolar macrophages. An overexpression of TIMP-2 has been shown to inhibit invasive and metastatic activity of tumor cells and decrease tumor growth in vivo[1]
Tissue inhibitors of metalloproteinases(基质金属蛋白酶抑制剂)	A family of secreted protease inhibitory proteins that regulates the activity of SECRETED MATRIX METALLOENDOPEPTIDASES. They play an important role in modulating the proteolysis of EXTRACELLULAR MATRIX, most notably during tissue remodeling and inflammatory processes[1]
Titubation(蹒跚)	Nodding movement of the head or body[2]
Titubation(蹒跚)	头或身体点头样动作[2]
Todds paralysis(Todd麻痹)	Todd's paralysis is a brief period of paralysis that occurs in the aftermath of a seizure[1]
TOF MRA(时间飞跃法MRA)	TOF MRA is a gradient echo sequence that depicts vascular flow by repeatedly applying a radio frequency (RF) pulse to a volume of tissue, followed by dephasing and rephasing gradients[1]

英文术语（中文术语）	定义（英文和/或中文）
Toll like receptors(Toll样受体)	A protein with a core domain composition consisting of a signal peptide, an extracellular domain with multiple Leucine rich repeat (Pfam:PF13855) domain (LRR), a cysteine-rich region, a single-pass transmembrane domain and a C-terminal cytoplasmic tail containing a TIR domain (Pfam:PF01582)[1]
Toronto Stroke Scale(多伦多中风量表)	The Toronto Stroke Scale was developed to assess neurologic deficit in acute stroke patients as part of a steroid therapy efficacy trial[1]
Torsion dystonia(扭转性肌张力障碍)	Sustained involuntary muscle contractions that produce twisting and repetitive movements of the body[2]
Torsion dystonia(扭转性肌张力障碍)	持续不自主的肌肉收缩引起身体的扭曲和重复的动作[2]
Torticollis(痉挛性斜颈)	Involuntary contractions of the "neck musculature" (FMA:71290) resulting in an abnormal posture of or abnormal movements of the head[2]
Torticollis(痉挛性斜颈)	颈部肌肉不自主收缩导致头部运动异常或位置异常[2]
transcortical aphasia(经皮质性失语)	Transcortical aphasia is characterized by a relative preservation of sentence repetition in the context of severe disturbances in the comprehension and/or production of oral language. It is divided into three types: transcortical motor, sensory and mixed aphasia[1]
Transcortical motor aphasia(经皮质运动性失语)	This is characterized by poor spontaneous speech but good repetition and comprehension. There is a variable naming deficit and the writing output is also poor. The localization of lesions is characteristically in the mesial frontal region or the supplementary speech area in the dominant hemisphere. These are often caused by an anterior cerebral artery stroke[1]
Transcortical sensory aphasia(经皮质感觉性失语)	This is characterized by fluent, semantic jargon, poor comprehension and good repetition. These patients usually have far more posterior lesions, usually in the watershed area between the middle cerebral and posterior cerebral circulation, although at times thalamic lesions are described with "transcortical sensory" features[1]

续　表

英文术语（中文术语）	定义（英文和/或中文）
Transcranial Doppler(经颅多普勒)	TCD ultrasound uses low frequency (2 MHz) pulsed sound to penetrate bony windows and visualize intracranial vessels of the circle of Willis. Its use has gained wide acceptance in stroke and neurologic intensive care units as a noninvasive means of assessing the patency of intracranial vessels[1]
Transforming growth factor beta(转化生长因子-β)	A factor synthesized in a wide variety of tissues. It acts synergistically with TGF-alpha in inducing phenotypic transformation and can also act as a negative autocrine growth factor. TGF-beta has a potential role in embryonal development, cellular differentiation, hormone secretion, and immune function. TGF-beta is found mostly as homodimer forms of separate gene products TGF-beta1, TGF-beta2 or TGF-beta3. Heterodimers composed of TGF-beta1 and 2 (TGF-beta1.2) or of TGF-beta2 and 3 (TGF-beta2.3) have been isolated. The TGF-beta proteins are synthesized as precursor proteins[1]
Transforming growth factor beta(转化生长因子-β)	TGF-β has an anti-inflammatory effect by inhibiting excessive neuroinflammation during the subacute phase of brain ischemia[1]
Transient ischemic attack(短暂性脑缺血发作)	A transient ischemic attack (TIA) is an episode in which neurological symptoms occur as a result of cerebrovascular disease, but resolve completely within 24 h[1]
Transthyretin(甲状腺素运载蛋白)	TTR, also known as prealbumin, is synthesized in the liver, in the choroid plexus and retina, and in the cytoplasm of ependymal cells of brain ventricles. It is a major plasma and CSF carrier of the thyroid hormone and retinol[1]
Treatment(治疗)	Used with diseases for therapeutic interventions except drug therapy, diet therapy, radiotherapy, and surgery, for which specific subheadings exist. The concept is also used for articles and books dealing with multiple therapies. [MeSH] [LIRADS] Intervention with the intent to slow the growth, cause necrosis, or resect from the liver an HCC. Examples include surgical resection, ablation, chemoembolization, radiation, and systemic chemotherapy[1]
Treatment of atherosclerotic cerebrovascular disease(动脉粥样硬化性脑血管病的治疗)	The goal of treatment of ischemic stroke is to restore blood flow to the affected area of the brain as quickly as possible, which means within the first hours after the stroke begins[1]

英文术语（中文术语）	定义（英文和/或中文）
Tremor(震颤)	An unintentional, oscillating to-and-fro muscle movement[2]
Tremor(震颤)	Tremor is exceptionally reported as an acute event in strokes. An acute resting tremor is reported in a patient with a lacunar infarction at the border between the thalamus and the internal capsule or lateral or posterior thalamus. Subthalamic infarcts can also be accompanied by an acute resting and action tremor[1]
Tremor(震颤)	一种无意的、振荡的肌肉往复运动[2]
Tremor by anatomical site(按解剖部位分类的震颤)	Tremor classified by the affected body part[2]
Tremor by anatomical site(按解剖部位分类的震颤)	按解剖部位分类的震颤[2]
Trial of ORG 10172 in acute stroke treatment(TOAST分型)	The TOAST (trial of ORG 10172 in acute stroke treatment) classification denotes five sub types of ischaemic stroke. large-artery atherosclerosis (embolus / thrombosis) cardioembolism (high-risk / medium-risk) small-vessel occlusion (lacune) stroke of other determined aetiology stroke of undetermined aetiology[1]
Triflusal(三氟柳)	Triflusal is an antiplatelet agent structurally related to aspirin that exerts its antithrombotic effect by acting on different targets involved in platelet aggregation and vascular inflammatory processes. In addition, triflusal increases nitric oxide synthesis in neutrophils, resulting in increased vasodilatory potential.8 Triflusal has already shown its efficacy in several thrombotic diseases[1]
Tritanomaly(蓝色弱)	Difficulty distinguishing between yellow and blue, possible related to dysfunction of the S photopigment[2]
Tritanomaly(蓝色弱)	黄色和蓝色区分障碍，可能是由于蓝色感光色素功能障碍所致[2]
Truncal ataxia(躯干性共济失调)	A kind of "ataxia" (HP:0001251) that affects the proximal musculature, especially that involved in gait stability[2]
Truncal ataxia(躯干性共济失调)	一种影响近端肌肉的共济失调（HP:0001251），尤其是那些参与步态稳定的肌肉[2]
Truncal titubation(躯干蹒跚)	Tremor of the trunk in an anterior-posterior plane at 3-4 Hz[2]
Truncal titubation(躯干蹒跚)	躯干在前-后平面以3-4 Hz的频率震颤[2]

续　表

英文术语（中文术语）	定义（英文和/或中文）
Truncular ataxia(闭合性共济失调)	Truncal ataxia is generally caused by midline damage to the cerebellar vermis and associated pathways. Patients with truncal ataxia may not be able to sit or stand without support. Truncal ataxia is a sign of ataxia characterized by instability of the trunk. It usually occurs during sitting [1]
Tuberothalamic artery infarction symptom(丘脑结节动脉梗死症状)	The tuberothalamic (or polar) artery arises from the PCoA and irrigates the anterior nuclei, the ventral anterior nucleus, amygdalofugal pathway, mamillothalamic tract, rostral part of the ventrolateral nucleus, ventral pole of the medial dorsal nucleus and ventral part of the internal medullary lamina [1]
Tumor necrosis factor alpha(肿瘤坏死因子a)	Serum glycoprotein produced by activated MACROPHAGES and other mammalian MONONUCLEAR LEUKOCYTES. It has necrotizing activity against tumor cell lines and increases ability to reject tumor transplants. Also known as TNF-alpha, it is only 30% homologous to TNF-beta (LYMPHOTOXIN), but they share TNF RECEPTORS [1]
Tumor necrosis factor beta(肿瘤坏死因子β)	A tumor necrosis factor family member that is released by activated LYMPHOCYTES. Soluble lymphotoxin is specific for TUMOR NECROSIS FACTOR RECEPTOR TYPE I; TUMOR NECROSIS FACTOR RECEPTOR TYPE II; and TUMOR NECROSIS FACTOR RECEPTOR SUPERFAMILY, MEMBER 14. Lymphotoxin-alpha can form a membrane-bound heterodimer with LYMPHOTOXIN-BETA that has specificity for the LYMPHOTOXIN BETA RECEPTOR [1]
Type I Hyperlipoproteinemia(高脂蛋白血症I型)	An inherited condition due to a deficiency of either LIPOPROTEIN LIPASE or APOLIPOPROTEIN C-II (a lipase-activating protein). The lack of lipase activities results in inability to remove CHYLOMICRONS and TRIGLYCERIDES from the blood which has a creamy top layer after standing [1]

续　表

英文术语（中文术语）	定义（英文和/或中文）
Type II Hyperlipoproteinemia(高脂蛋白血症II型)	Hypercholesterolemia that is caused by mutation in the LOW DENSITY LIPOPROTEIN RECEPTOR gene. This receptor defect prevents LDL binding to the cell membrane and uptake of cholesterol which normally suppresses further cholesterol synthesis. A group of familial disorders characterized by elevated circulating cholesterol contained in either LOW-DENSITY LIPOPROTEINS alone or also in VERY-LOW-DENSITY LIPOPROTEINS (pre-beta lipoproteins). Type Ⅱ b hyperlipoproteinemia is caused by mutation in the receptor-binding domain of APOLIPOPROTEIN B-100 which is a major component of LOW-DENSITY LIPOPROTEINS and VERY-LOW-DENSITY LIPOPROTEINS resulting in reduced clearance of these lipoproteins. It is characterized by both hypercholesterolemia and HYPERTRIGLYCERIDEMIA (combined hyperlipidemia)[1]
Type III Hyperlipoproteinemia(高脂蛋白血症III型)	An autosomal recessively inherited disorder characterized by the accumulation of intermediate-density lipoprotein (IDL or broad-beta-lipoprotein). IDL has a CHOLESTEROL to TRIGLYCERIDES ratio greater than that of VERY-LOW-DENSITY LIPOPROTEINS. This disorder is due to mutation of APOLIPOPROTEINS E, a receptor-binding component of VLDL and CHYLOMICRONS, resulting in their reduced clearance and high plasma levels of both cholesterol and triglycerides[1]
Type IV Hyperlipoproteinemia(高脂蛋白血症IV型)	A hypertriglyceridemia disorder, often with autosomal dominant inheritance. It is characterized by the persistent elevations of plasma TRIGLYCERIDES, endogenously synthesized and contained predominantly in VERY-LOW-DENSITY LIPOPROTEINS (pre-beta lipoproteins). In contrast, the plasma CHOLESTEROL and PHOSPHOLIPIDS usually remain within normal limits[1]

英文术语（中文术语）	定义（英文和/或中文）
Type V Hyperlipoproteinemia(高脂蛋白血症 V 型)	A severe type of hyperlipidemia, sometimes familial, that is characterized by the elevation of both plasma CHYLOMICRONS and TRIGLYCERIDES contained in VERY-LOW-DENSITY LIPOPROTEINS. Type V hyperlipoproteinemia is often associated with DIABETES MELLITUS and is not caused by reduced LIPOPROTEIN LIPASE activity as in HYPERLIPOPROTEINEMIA TYPE I [1]
Ubiquitin fusion degradation protein(泛素融合降解蛋白)	Ubiquitin fusion degradation protein (UFDP) is an enzyme in the ubiquitin degradation pathway that is expressed in many body tissue types [1]
Unilateral deafness(单耳聋)	Sudden unilateral hearing loss with vertigo frequently occurs with anterior inferior cerebellar artery occlusion proximal to the internal auditory artery [1]
Unilateral ptosis(单侧上睑下垂)	A "unilateral" (PATO:0000634) form of ptosis [2]
Unilateral ptosis(单侧上睑下垂)	发生于一只眼（PATO:0000634）的上睑下垂 [2]
Upbeat nystagmus(上跳性眼震)	In primary position the Upbeat nystagmus beats upward. The associated oscillopsias are often very irritating, but the symptoms are usually transient [2]
Upbeat nystagmus(上跳性眼震)	此型眼球震颤呈眼球跳动上升。震动幻视通常非常严重，但是症状通常是短暂的 [2]
Upper limb postural tremor(上肢姿势性震颤)	A type of tremors that is triggered by holding an arm in a fixed position [2]
Upper limb postural tremor(上肢姿势性震颤)	一种将手臂固定在某个特殊位置而诱发的震颤 [2]
Upper quadrantanopsia without cognitive impairment(无认知障碍的上象限盲)	A rarer but typical presentation of AChA infarcts is the triad of contralateral severe hemiparesis, hemihypesthesia and upper quadrantanopsia or contralateral versus ipsilateral hemianopsia (in the case of lateral geniculate body or optic tract, respectively) without cognitive disturbances, in contrast with MCA infarction [1]
Upper quadrantanopsia without cognitive impairment(无认知障碍的上象限盲)	Loss of vision in a quarter section of the visual field of one or both eyes; if bilateral, it may be homonymous or heteronymous, binasal or bitemporal, or crossed, for example, involving the upper quadrant in one eye and the lower quadrant in the other [1]

续　表

英文术语（中文术语）	定义（英文和/或中文）
Urinalysis(尿常规)	Examination of urine by chemical, physical, or microscopic means. Routine urinalysis usually includes performing chemical screening tests, determining specific gravity, observing any unusual color or odor, screening for bacteriuria, and examining the sediment microscopically[1]
Vascular cell adhesion molecule 1(血管细胞黏附分子1)	Cytokine-induced cell adhesion molecule present on activated endothelial cells, tissue macrophages, dendritic cells, bone marrow fibroblasts, myoblasts, and myotubes. It is important for the recruitment of leukocytes to sites of inflammation. (From Pigott & Power, The Adhesion Molecule FactsBook, 1993, p.154)[1]
Vascular disorder(血管性疾病)	Vascular disease is an abnormal condition of the blood vessels. Blood vessels (arteries and veins) are the tubes through which blood is pumped throughout the body[1]
Vascular parkinsonism(血管性帕金森综合征)	Acute ischemic infarction of the caudate, putamen, globus pallidus, or brain stem can result in parkinsonism. Parkinsonism of vascular origin is a controversial entity. Only 2% of patients with cerebral infarcts may have a parkinsonian syndrome[1]
Vasovagal syncope(血管迷走神经性晕厥)	Loss of consciousness due to a reduction in blood pressure that is associated with an increase in vagal tone and peripheral vasodilation[2]
Vasovagal syncope(血管迷走神经性晕厥)	由于血压降低伴随的迷走神经张力和周围血管扩张增加从而导致的意识丧失[2]
Vegetable(蔬菜)	cruciferous and green leafy vegetables (e.g. cabbages, turnips, broccoli), together with citrus fruit and juice, protected against stroke[1]
Vegetable(蔬菜)	dietary practice of completely avoiding meat products in the diet[1]
Venous thromboembolism(静脉栓塞)	Embolism of a vein by an embolus carried in a direction opposite to that of the normal blood current, after being diverted into a smaller vein[1]
Venous thrombosis(静脉血栓形成)	The formation of a blood clot (thrombus) in the lumen of a vein. It has many genetic and acquired risk factors[1]

续 表

英文术语（中文术语）	定义（英文和/或中文）
Vertebral artery dissection(椎动脉夹层)	Vertebral artery dissection is a dissection (a flap-like tear) of the inner lining of the vertebral artery, which is located in the neck and supplies blood to the brain[1]
Vertebral artery infarction symptom(椎动脉梗死症状)	The vertebral arteries give origin to two arteries before joining to form the basilar artery: the anterior spinal artery, which supplies the medial medulla oblongata and the upper cervical cord, and the PICA, which supplies the inferior cerebellum and the dorsolateral medulla[1]
Vertebrobasilar dolichoectasia(椎基底动脉延长扩张症)	Vertebrobasilar dolichoectasia (VBD) is an arteriopathy characterized by distinct dilatation, elongation and tortuosity of the basilar artery (BA) and the vertebral artery (VA). It is an uncommon vasculopathy of unclear aetiology affecting the arterial wall of vertebral and/or basilar arteries, which is easily misdiagnosed[1]
Vertebrobasilar infarction syndrome(椎基底动脉梗死综合征)	The posterior circulation is also called the vertebrobasilar circulation. The two vertebral arteries leave the subclavian arteries, pass through transverse foramina in the apophysis of the sixth to the second cervical vertebra, enter the cranium through the foramen magnum, and join together to form the basilar artery (BA)[1]
Vertical gaze paresis(垂直注视麻痹)	Voluntary or reflex vertical gaze (tested by oculocephalic and caloric maneuvers and Bell phenomenon) is often abolished. One or both eyes may rest in a downward position. Isolated paralysis of upward or downward gaze occurs less frequently. In human patients with vertical gaze paralysis due to vascular disease, bilateral lesions are found in the midbrain tegmentum[1]
Vertical nystagmus(垂直性眼震)	Vertical nystagmus may present with either up-beating or down-beating eye movements or both. When present in the straight-ahead position of gaze it is referred to as upbeat nystagmus or downbeat nystagmus[2]
Vertical nystagmus(垂直性眼震)	垂直眼球震颤可出现向上跳动或向下跳动或两者兼有的眼球运动。当出现在凝视的正前方位置它被称为向上震颤或向下眼球震颤[2]
Vertigo(眩晕)	An abnormal sensation of spinning while the body is actually stationary[2]

英文术语（中文术语）	定义（英文和/或中文）
Vertigo(眩晕)	Vertigo is an unpleasant distortion of static gravitational orientation or an erroneous perception of motion of either the sufferer or the environment. It is not a well-defined disease entity, but rather the outcome of many pathological processes causing a mismatch between the visual, vestibular, and somatosensory systems, all of which subserve both static and dynamic spatial orientation. Physiological and clinical vestibular vertigo syndromes are commonly characterized by a combination of phenomena involving perceptual, ocular motor, postural and vegetative manifestations: vertigo, nystagmus, ataxia and nausea. The vertigo itself results from a disturbance of cortical spatial orientation, while nystagmus and ocular deviations are secondary to a direction-specific imbalance in the vestibulo-ocular reflex. Postural imbalance and vestibular ataxia are caused by inappropriate or abnormal inactivation of vestibulospinal pathways. Unpleasant vegetative effects, such as nausea and vomiting, are related to clinical activation of the medullary vomiting centre [1]
Vertigo(眩晕)	身体静止不动却自觉旋转的异常感觉 [2]
Very low density lipoprotein Cholesterol(极低密度脂蛋白胆固醇)	Cholesterol which is contained in or bound to very low density lipoproteins (VLDL). High circulating levels of VLDL cholesterol are found in HYPERLIPOPROTEINEMIA TYPE IIB. The cholesterol on the VLDL is eventually delivered by LOW-DENSITY LIPOPROTEINS to the tissues after the catabolism of VLDL to INTERMEDIATE-DENSITY LIPOPROTEINS, then to LDL [1]
Vestibular nystagmus(前庭性眼震)	Nystagmus due to disturbance of the vestibular system; eye movements are rhythmic, with slow and fast components [2]
Vestibular nystagmus(前庭性眼震)	眼球震颤由于前庭系统的干扰;眼球运动的节奏，用慢速和快速的组件 [2]
Visinin like protein 1(视锥蛋白样蛋白-1)	Visinin-like protein (VLP)-1 is the human homolog of a protein that was identified by screening mice with gene-array analyses for biomarkers that are preferentially and abundantly produced in brain [1]

续　表

英文术语（中文术语）	定义（英文和/或中文）
Visual agnosia(视觉失认)	Visual agnosia denotes impaired recognition of visually presented material in a patient with normal or almost normal visual acuity; auditory and tactile recognition is normally spared. The term visual agnosia was introduced in 1891 by Sigmund Freud and it stresses the role of internally represented knowledge in visual perception[1]
Visual field defect(视野缺损)	Visual field defect[2]
Visual field defect(视野缺损)	Visual field defects indicate involvement of the visual pathways and the pattern of visual field defects help in localizing site of the lesion. Visual field defects in the affected eye at presentation included diffuse visual field loss (48%), altitudinal defects (15%), central or cecocentral scotoma (8.3%), arcuate or double arcuate (4.5%), hemianopic defects (4.2%), and others[1]
Visual field defect(视野缺损)	部分或全部视野的缺损[2]
Visual hallucinations(视幻觉)	A kind of hallucination,which can see the image of a simple form. pathological illusion,if when awareness is clear which is more common in schizophrenia, while in the sense of disturbance occurs, which is more common in delirium or hazy state[2]
Visual hallucinations(视幻觉)	幻觉的一种。可以看到简单不成形的形象，病理性幻视如在意识清晰时出现，多见于精神分裂症，如在意识障碍时出现，则多见于谵妄状态或朦胧状态[2]
Visual impairment(视觉障碍)	Limitation in visual functions. Visual impairments limiting one or more of the basic functions of the eye: visual acuity, dark adaptation, color vision, or peripheral vision. These may result from EYE DISEASES; OPTIC NERVE DISEASES; VISUAL PATHWAY diseases; OCCIPITAL LOBE diseases; OCULAR MOTILITY DISORDERS; and other conditions (From Newell, Ophthalmology: Principles and Concepts, 7th ed, p132)[1]
Vitamin B intake(维生素B摄入量)	There is a positive correlation between homocysteine levels and stroke. For this reason, guidelines on the primary prevention of stroke recommend the use of B vitamins in patients with known elevated homocysteine levels[1]

英文术语（中文术语）	定义（英文和/或中文）
Vitamin D intake(维生素 D 摄入量)	Higher intake of vitamin D (≥600 IU/d) was associated with a lower incidence of coronary heart disease and stroke, in men but not in women[1]
Vitamin E intake(维生素 E 摄入量)	Vitamin E is a lipid-soluble antioxidant that increases the resistance of LDL cholesterol to oxidation, reduces proliferation of smooth muscle cells, and reduces adhesiveness of platelets to collagen. This vitamin inhibits lipid peroxidation by scavenging reactive oxygen species and preserving cell membranes[1]
Voice tremor(声音震颤)	A wavering, unsteady voice that reflects involuntary and approximately sinusoidal oscillation of motor unit firings of laryngeal muscles. Vocal tremor results in low frequency modulations of voice frequency or amplitude and intermittent voice instability[2]
Voice tremor(声音震颤)	一个摇摆不定、不稳定的声音，反映喉肌的运动单位不自主的正弦振荡。声音震颤导致声音频率或幅度的低频调制和间歇性的声音不稳定[2]
Vomiting(呕吐)	Forceful ejection of the contents of the stomach through the mouth by means of a series of involuntary spasmic contractions[2]
Vomiting(呕吐)	通过一系列无意识的痉挛收缩而使胃内容物经口有力地喷出[2]
von Willebrand factor(血管性假血友病因子)	A high-molecular-weight plasma protein, produced by endothelial cells and megakaryocytes, that is part of the factor VIII/von Willebrand factor complex. The von Willebrand factor has receptors for collagen, platelets, and ristocetin activity as well as the immunologically distinct antigenic determinants. It functions in adhesion of platelets to collagen and hemostatic plug formation. The prolonged bleeding time in VON WILLEBRAND DISEASES is due to the deficiency of this factor[1]

续　表

英文术语（中文术语）	定义（英文和/或中文）
Wallenberg syndrome(延髓背外侧综合征)	The laterodorsal medullary stroke is the most common of those three syndromes and is named the Wallenberg syndrome, after Adolf Wallenberg (1862–1946), a German neurologist. Wallenberg syndrome and an infarct in the inferior cerebellum stroke can be seen in isolation or together, the latter being usually the case if the vertebral artery is occluded[1]
Warfarin(华法林)	Warfarin, a coumarin derivative, produces an anticoagulant effect by interfering with the cyclic interconversion of vitamin K and its 2,3 epoxide (vitamin K epoxide). Vitamin K is a cofactor for the carboxylation of glutamate residues to γ-carboxyglutamates (Gla) on the N-terminal regions of vitamin K–dependent proteins[1]
Watershed infarction syndrome(分水岭梗死综合征)	Watershed (or borderzone) infarcts represent about 5% of all strokes. They involve the junction of distal regions of two arterial systems. WS infarcts have been studied best in the anterior circulation in relationship to severe stenosis or occlusion of the ICA. Two typical patterns are observed: cortical WS (CWS) and the internal WS (IWS) strokes. The CWS area is located superficially in the cortex between the MCA, ACA and PCA territories. Strokes appear radiologically as wedges extending from the prefrontal or parieto-occipital cortex down to the frontal and occipital horns of the lateral ventricle respectively. The IWS area is situated in an anterior–posterior orientation in the centrum semiovale and along the lateral ventricle[1]
Weber syndrome［韦伯氏综合征(大脑脚综合征)］	Weber syndrome is a midbrain stroke syndrome that involves the fascicles of the oculomotor nerve resulting in an ipsilateral CN III palsy and contralateral hemiplegia or hemiparesis. Using imaging alone, it is difficult to distinguish Weber from Benedikt syndrome, unless clear involvement of the red nucleus can be identified[1]
Wernicke's aphasia(Wernicke失语)	This is characterized by fluent, paraphasic speech with impaired comprehension, repetition, and naming. Neologistic jargon output is distinctive and occurs in severe Wernicke's aphasia, associated with lesions of both the superior temporal and inferior parietal regions[1]

英文术语（中文术语）	定义（英文和/或中文）
Western Aphasia Battery(西方失语症成套测验)	The Western Aphasia Battery is a comprehensive test of language function for individuals with aphasia and aged 18–89 years. Test administration time is 30–60 min, depending on the severity of the patient's aphasia and coexisting deficits (e.g., apraxia, dysarthria). As stated in the test manual, the aim of the WAB is to "evaluate the main clinical aspects of language function, content, fluency, auditory comprehension, repetition, naming, reading, writing, and calculations." The WAB is designed to test all language modalities: reading, writing, listening, speaking, and gestural communication. The WAB-R has the same overall structure as the original WAB and also includes supplementary tests of reading and writing of irregular words and nonwords, and a bedside screening test that takes approximately 15 min to administer[1]
Wolf Motor Function Test(Wolf运动功能测试)	he original version of the Wolf Motor Function Test (WMFT) was developed by Wolf et al to examine the effects of constraint-induced movement therapy (CIMT) for survivors of stroke and traumatic brain injury. The original form of the test consisted of 21 simple tasks sequenced according to joints involved (shoulder to fingers) and level of difficulty (gross to fine motor skill)[1]
Writer's cramp(书写痉挛)	A focal dystonia of the fingers, hand, and/or forearm that appears when the affected person attempts to do a task that requires fine motor movements such as writing or playing a musical instrument[2]
Writer's cramp(书写痉挛)	手指、手和/或前臂的局灶性肌张力障碍，在受影响的人试图完成需要精细动作的任务时出现，如书写或玩乐器的任务出[2]